ABO...

Jane Benn... ... ... work to p... ... ...reer ... ...ounselling, teaching and ...ing in the field of natural fertility management after experiencing the revelations of charting her own cycle in the mid-eighties. Jane also facilitates workshops for girls and their mums celebrating their approaching menarche and fertility, and for dads on how to handle the changes and stay close to their daughters. The author of *A Blessing Not a Curse* (Sally Milner Publishing, 2002) and co-author of *The Natural Fertility Management Kits for Contraception* and *Conception* (NFMKits, 2004) with Francesca Naish, Jane has a daughter and three stepsons and lives with her husband in Central Victoria amongst 500-million-year-old granite boulders. She enjoys standing on her head, pulling out weeds and making felt animals, but not all at once.

Alexandra Pope has a background in education and since 1988 has worked in private practice as a psychotherapist and more recently as a coach. Based on her experiences of working with women and girls and the discovery of the value of her own cycle, Alexandra has been running workshops and lecturing in Australia and the UK on the power of the cycle for women's creative, psychological and physical wellbeing since 1993. She is currently developing a women's leadership program based on this work. Alexandra is the author of *The Wild Genie* (Sally Milner Publishing, 2001) and *The Woman's Quest* (Self published, 2006).

Passionate, articulate and slightly driven, Alexandra has the wild idea that women everywhere will one day experience their menstrual cycle as a really cool, empowering process—an intrinsic, healthy and dynamic part of their being that they simply love to have.

THE
PILL

THE PILL

Are you *sure* it's for you?

JANE BENNETT AND ALEXANDRA POPE

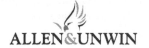

ALLEN&UNWIN

Allen & Unwin
83 Alexander Street
Crows Nest NSW 2065
Australia
Phone: (61 2) 8425 0100
Fax: (61 2) 9906 2218
Email: info@allenandunwin.com
Web: www.allenandunwin.com

The Cataloguing-in-Publication entry is available
from the National Library of Australia.

ISBN 978 1 74175 079 9

Text design by Nada Backovic Designs
Set in 10.5/14 pt Ehrhardt by Midland Typesetters, Australia
Printed in Australia by McPherson's Printing Group

10 9 8 7 6 5 4 3 2 1

AUTHORS' NOTE

The content of this book is intended for guidance only. We are not medical practitioners—the information and suggestions we make are not meant to be prescriptive. Any attempt to treat a medical condition should always come under the direction of a qualified health practitioner, preferably one experienced in nutrition and naturopathic methods. Neither the authors nor the publisher accept responsibility for any consequences of a reader failing to take appropriate medical advice.

CONTENTS

Appendices

INTRODUCTION

The promise of an effective contraceptive pill has been an irresistible convenience for a great many women over the last half century. With more than 300 million of us worldwide having at some time been on the Pill and a hundred million plus currently taking it, the Pill is clearly a very popular drug.

If you're fertile, sexually active and at a stage of life when you don't want babies, or more babies, or not just yet anyway, then the issue of contraception is a BIG one. You don't want to get pregnant, you'd rather not face an abortion and you may be willing to make compromises just to feel secure. With a feeling of security about your contraception it's easier to relax and enjoy your sex life.

The Pill, as a vehicle for us to 'make love not babies', has undoubtedly been part of our collective evolution and has allowed us to explore our sexuality and sexual relationships with greater freedom than ever before. Like the Kylie, Diana or Madonna of pharmaceuticals, the Pill became an icon soon after its release in the early sixties. Heralded as one of the great inventions of the twentieth century, the catalyst of the sexual revolution and the technological enabler of women's liberation, the Pill is now often thought of as a synonym for contraception itself. However, much as we may wish it, the Pill is *not* the perfect contraception—not as effective, not as convenient and certainly not the boon to sexuality that popular wisdom would have us believe.

The first oral contraceptive commercially available was Enovid. It was approved by the US Food and Drug Administration on the basis of a small clinical study that involved 132 Puerto Rican women who took the Pill for a year. Three women, who were both young and fertile, died during the study after severe chest pains. No autopsy was performed. They were simply eliminated from the study.[1]

By the end of 1961, a year after its release, Enovid's manufacturer had on record many cases of thrombosis and embolism in women taking Enovid. Among these were eleven deaths. Nonetheless, even as evidence grew of these and other problems, the hopes for the Pill were such that most of the medical and scientific community valiantly tried to still the growing storm.

At this time Nobel Laureate Frederick Robbins, speaking at a meeting of the American Association of Medical Colleges, said, 'The dangers of overpopulation are so great that we may have to use certain techniques of conception control that may entail considerable risk to the individual woman'.[2] It was clear by 1969, however, that the Pill was 'saving the saved' in that its most loyal users were middle-class women from developed countries, who had, by and large, been controlling their fertility successfully for decades anyway, well before the arrival of the Pill.

While the developing world may not have embraced this new drug, the vast commercial potential of the Pill was quickly recognised by pharmaceutical companies and heavily promoted to doctors and women alike. In the 1960s the Pill was presented as the modern way for a woman to manage her fertility. When it became impossible to ignore the dangers of the early Pills, new 'low dose' formulations were released in 1975. This measure reduced some of the earlier problems but not others, nonetheless these new generation Pills were heralded as 'safe'.

For young women exploring their contraceptive choices today, the Pill is often presented as the only responsible way to manage their fertility. It's also widely used for all manner of other conditions, complaints and conveniences—from skin problems and irregular cycles to period-free exams and honeymoons. A recent study found that nine out of ten American women have taken the Pill at some time and around one-third are current users. A similar pattern of use is repeated throughout the Western world and it's becoming a more acceptable and accessible form of contraception in other countries as well. As the Pill is most often taken long term, as if for a chronic condition—in this case fertility—we can see how it's achieved the status of the world's most widely used drug.

The Oral Contraceptive Pill is obviously taken as a pill by mouth. However, for the purposes of this book we take the liberty of using the term 'the Pill' to cover hormonal contraception generally, all of which are means of delivering synthetic oestrogen and progesterone, or synthetic progesterone alone, to a woman's body. Where necessary we distinguish one from another, as in implants, injections, rings or patches. Otherwise we simply use the term 'the Pill'.

In *The Pill* we seek to unpack the myths and realities about the Pill, and consider its influence on sexuality, fertility, relationships and physical and psychological health. We endeavour to give you the tools to become your own expert so you can find the most appropriate contraception for you, as you explore the depths and pleasures of your sexuality and enjoy menstrual wellbeing.

The Pill, by its hormonal action, impacts profoundly on all our organs and bodily systems in order to have its effect on our fertility. Drawing from scientific research and the experiences of real women, we examine the considerable, and often vastly under-acknowledged, side-effects of the Pill—from depression and loss of libido to brittle bones and cancer. We consider the consequences of interfering with our natural cycles and rhythms, and explore the somewhat radical idea that the menstrual cycle may be intrinsic to women's physical and psychological health—during our years of natural cycling—without which we may be seriously impoverished.

We challenge the perception that the Pill has been a great boon to relationships. We look at the hormonal fallout from the Pill, the issue of contraception in relationships and how this impacts on both men and women. As contraception is of central concern for heterosexuals for much of their fertile lives, or the fertile life of a couple, when we write about 'relationships' in this book, we're referring to those of a male-female gender mix, for obvious reasons.

In *The Pill* we also look at alternatives to chemical contraception and what they have to offer, as well as understanding success rates and how you can make them work for you. We outline practical steps that you can follow to ensure contraceptive cover, speedy return of cycles if you come off the Pill, and how you can achieve good menstrual health. You'll read about the benefits of having a variety of contraceptive methods available so you can make the most appropriate choices according to your particular circumstances and needs.

You've probably noticed by now that we're not subscribers to the view that the Pill is *the* modern contraception. In fact, we have grave reservations on many fronts, which come from long and careful investigation of scientific research, listening to women's experiences of the Pill, as well as our own exploration of fertility cycles and helping women to learn about theirs. The latter has revealed to us a surprisingly rich feminine experience, and one that no woman, having discovered, would wish to give up for the Pill, especially while other methods of contraception are available.

By understanding the myths and the truths about the Pill, you'll be able to see more clearly what it can offer you and what it can't. By considering the range of contraception available, you can make choices according to your particular contraceptive needs, health and lifestyle. This is true informed choice and we hope that by writing this book we have been able to contribute to your understanding so that you can freely choose what will best suit you.

CHAPTER 1

ARE YOU CONFUSED? YOU'RE NOT ALONE!

Are you busy and just want a quick reliable contraception? Do you want birth control that's easy to understand and use? Do you get confused about what you need to do for effective contraception as well as how you can best protect yourself from sexually transmitted diseases?

If you're on the Pill did you go on it for skin or period problems? Or are you taking it for contraception? Are you in a relationship and pregnancy is just not an option? Would you like a relationship and are on the Pill just in case?

Or are you thinking about going on the Pill wondering if it's as effective as they say? Do you want to know what the side-effects may be?

Do you want to know more about how your body works and how contraception will affect you? Do you worry about interfering with your fertility or your menstrual cycle? And if you don't go on the Pill what else is there?

This book will help you to figure out what's right for *you*. Decisions about contraception are really important, so it's worth exploring your options.

You're fertile for many years and by choosing the right contraception method or methods that work for you, you are more likely to find the best fit for your lifestyle, values and goals. Naturally, this will be different from person to person. The more you know and understand about contraception and your own body the more you're able to tailor the methods you use to suit you. Then you can relax and enjoy your sex life.

A not so happy choice

Often we end up on the Pill because it seems the most obvious thing to do as a teenager. Kim was just starting to explore her sexuality at eighteen and in her second year of college and she wanted to do the 'responsible thing' so she went on the Pill. It was almost a rite of passage and so easy. She explained to the doctor what she wanted and five minutes later she had a prescription. She doesn't remember hearing anything about possible disadvantages or health issues—just 'use a condom as well' and instructions on 'what to do if she forgot to take the Pill'. If she'd known about the consequences she may still have taken the Pill for a little while, but not for almost twenty years.

I had so much going for me and yet was so sad, so often. Now I know my natural state is happiness, not moody depression from artificial hormones.

KIM, 37

At the time she went on the Pill it made Kim feel like an adult. It offered her regular 'periods', cleared her acne, freed her from pain during the first day or so of her period, and gave her birth control. Later, as a career woman, the Pill still seemed to offer Kim great convenience. Every time she visited the doctor to renew the script, she was told she shouldn't smoke and take the Pill but never about the side-effects she may suffer.

During her twenties and thirties, Kim found it difficult to lose weight, had monthly migraines, very little sex drive and felt chronically low. She just thought it was *her*. 'Why wasn't I happy? I had so much going for me and yet was so sad, so often. I didn't realise the Pill was making me depressed,' she admits. 'I thought my blue moods were just part of my psychological make-up.'

Kim decided to come off the Pill when she heard a talk about its side-effects. To her dismay she realised *all* her main health problems were known side-effects of the Pill. At 37, she had taken the Pill for almost twenty years, and finally felt the confidence to stop.

What a surprise. In the first week after she stopped taking the Pill Kim felt a lot of anger, partly because she had suffered side-effects from the Pill for so long without knowing the cause. This was also due to her liver detoxing after years of processing the synthetic hormones in the Pill. All drugs taken orally are first delivered to the liver before entering general circulation and years of a daily Pill is a considerable toxic load for this vital organ. With the support of her naturopath she was able to restore her health and hormonal balance. After two weeks she began to feel like a new woman—'I was amazed. I woke in the morning feeling refreshed, awake and alive. I felt light and vibrant—a feeling of happiness and an absence from depression that I was very unfamiliar with. It would seem that my natural state is happiness, not moody depression from artificial hormones.'

Women taking the Pill were almost twice as likely to be depressed, compared to those not on the Pill.

Kim's menstrual cycle is still irregular and she suspects this will take some time to return to balance. But her migraines have gone and she's enjoying a wonderful resurgence in her sex drive. Kim now likes getting her period and being able to read her body's signs of fertility and know when she's fertile if she wants to get pregnant.

It was only after she stopped taking the Pill that Kim's mother confessed that she had also had bad migraines while on the Pill, but hadn't made the connection between her own experience and Kim's.

The next step Kim took was to quit smoking. At first she found experiencing her natural hormonal cycle and managing her emotions without smoking was challenging, 'However, I feel like I'm becoming closer to my real self,' she reflects. 'I am happier and feel healthier and relieved. I had no idea what it meant to be a natural woman. I think information about fertility awareness should be mandatory. If I'd learnt all this in high school it would certainly have saved me a lot of trouble.'

> All her main health problems were known side-effects of the Pill.

From powerless to empowered

Lisa's experience on the Pill echoes many women's stories. Like so many she struggled with various forms of birth control, never feeling right with them, until she finally learnt about fertility awareness, and that changed everything.

As a responsible sixteen-year-old, she went on the Pill before having sex with her boyfriend. After a few years of hating the Pill, especially the weight gain, she switched to an IUD. For over six years it worked well enough apart from the heavy menstrual bleeding and cramps.

One summer she had her IUD removed while her boyfriend was away, and didn't get a new one put in until after his return. In that brief window she got pregnant. Neither of them was ready for a child, as they were both in the middle of their degrees, so Lisa had an abortion. She was pressured to go back on the Pill—pitched as the most effec-

> Often we end up on the Pill because it seems the most obvious thing to do as a teenager.

tive method of contraception—and was freaked out enough to agree, even though it didn't fit with her healthy lifestyle. After only a few months, she rebelled. 'I felt horrible on the Pill,' she recalls. 'I had perpetual PMS. I felt sluggish and heavy, cranky and unsexy.'

After graduating from university, she had a prolonged and rocky break-up with her boyfriend, and moved to the city to start her career. She made do with condoms during the few brief affairs she had during that time.

Lisa's life was transformed when she started seeing a fertility awareness counsellor. She had always recorded her periods on a calendar and was fascinated by being able to identify ovulation. 'I was a perfect candidate for fertility awareness,' she admits. 'I was fed up with artificial birth control. I was single and not sexually active in the early learning days. I was motivated to become healthy and more in tune with my body's natural rhythms.'

By the time she met her future husband Lisa was confident enough to use her charts to determine her fertile and infertile days and plan their dates accordingly. Lisa felt her life and options so dramatically changed by fertility awareness that she studied to become a fertility awareness teacher.

I felt horrible on the Pill. I had perpetual PMS. I felt sluggish and heavy, cranky and unsexy.

LISA, 43

Ready to start a family

Catherine had used the Pill for contraception most of the time since she was seventeen years old. When she was 35 she and her husband Rob were ready to start a family. They had always planned to have children and wanted to be financially set up so they could manage on one income while the children were little. The time had finally come. So, Catherine went off the Pill. As the months went by she became more and more alarmed. Her cycles were all over the place. The longest was 75 days, the shortest was 34 days and they were totally unpredictable. And, Catherine wasn't getting pregnant.

Fourteen months later, hearing her fertility clock ticking loudly, Catherine and Rob sought professional help. They found that Catherine's hormone levels were completely out of balance—her oestrogen was very low, and her luteinising hormone was very high relative to her follicle-stimulating hormone. She also had very little cervical mucus, which is crucial for a successful passage of sperm to egg.

Catherine received naturopathic treatment for her hormone levels. Both she and Rob went onto a good pre-conception healthcare program so they'd be in optimum reproductive and general health for when the time came to conceive their baby. It took five months for Catherine's cycles to become regular and a few more months for them to conceive. The pregnancy went well and Catherine gave birth to a beautiful little boy. Now, two and a half years later, they're awaiting the arrival of a little brother or sister for Nicholas.

While she'll never know for sure, Catherine strongly suspects that all her years of taking the Pill were the reason her hormone levels were so out of whack. She never went on the Pill again and she and Rob success-fully used a combination of barrier and fertility awareness methods for contraception between their babies.

During my 30 years in practice, I have seen countless women and girls who experience major menstrual, reproductive and general health problems when they come off the Pill—problems that weren't evident prior to its use. Quite frequently these conditions then go on to threaten future fertility.

FRANCESCA NAISH, NATUROPATH

CHAPTER 2

THE PILL IS A DRUG

The Pill is a unique drug in that it's designed to interfere with one of your normal bodily functions—with fertility itself—and is the only prescription drug used long term that does so. Different to all other drugs the Pill is taken by healthy young women whose only problem is their fertility. While it's often used for menstrual problems the Pill wasn't initially designed to deal with these kinds of health issues.

The Pill is said to be the most commonly used drug of all, taken at some time by more than 300 million women worldwide. Currently about 100 million women take this drug every day and tens of millions are using injections, implants and other forms of chemical contraception.

It's interesting to note that when the Pill was first made available manufacturers told women and doctors it was safe. They were soon shown to be wrong, and now we hear that, yes, the original high-dose Pills were problematic and unsafe but that current formulations are totally fine. Does this reflect genuine concern for women's health or is it just marketing?

He offered me medication for the migraines, which seemed ridiculous to me because they were due to the Pill. Why take more drugs to counteract the side-effects of another? His last comment was, 'You'll have to go back on the Pill eventually.'

JENNIFER, 33

The arrival of the Pill

We know that couples have actively limited the size of their families for thousands of years. Our ancestors used abstinence, prolonged breast-feeding, withdrawal, douches, sponges soaked in various household substances, local herbs and plants, imagination and ingenuity. In fact, contraceptive practices predate even agriculture.

A major shift to manufactured methods of contraception began in 1843, when Charles Goodyear (yes! as in the tyres) and Thomas Hancock developed the process for vulcanising rubber. Condoms could be mass-produced[1] and a few decades later the rubber diaphragm was developed and also became popular. In addition a whole array of devices, creams, pessaries, douches and literature about contraception became available and a significant decline in infant mortality made it all the more neces-sary to limit family size.

However, this all took place in an atmosphere dominated by per-sistent Victorian taboos around *anything* to do with sex. With severe legal, religious and medical limitations placed on contraception the success of birth control in the decades up to the middle of the twentieth century was a testimony to the will of those needing contraception.[2] Many pharmacies didn't sell contraceptives until well into the 1950s and 1960s, and even then restricted sales to only those customers who were verifiably married. Until 1965 it was illegal in the state of Connecticut for even married couples to use contraceptives![3]

During the 1960s a sexual revolution took place and contraception became much more easily available. Both men and women began to feel able to explore their sexuality outside the confines of marriage, and effec-tive, safe contraception came to be seen as a universal right. The Pill, when it became available in 1960 in the US and 1961 in Australia and the UK, did indeed cause a massive switch in the *type* of contraception people used. It brought a major shift of emphasis with women taking greater, or sole, responsibility for contraception. Nonetheless family size didn't change that much.

At the same time the attitude of doctors towards contraception changed dramatically. Where many had previously been ambivalent about contraception, being able to prescribe the Pill made all the difference and contraception has largely become the prerogative of the medical profession ever since.

There were enormous problems with the higher dose pills available up to 1975, with blood clots causing strokes, amputations, permanent disability and death at the top of the list. Nonetheless it took considerable pressure from concerned doctor and consumer groups to have these problems acknowledged and warnings placed inside Pill packets. Current medical research on women who have at any time used the Pill makes a clear distinction between those who took it before 1975 and those who didn't.

However, current third-generation oral contraceptives still have considerable side-effects and many are cumulative as the nutritional disturbances caused by the Pill's effect on our processing of nutrients gathers momentum over time. Many studies have found that these newer Pills have actually increased the risk of thrombosis. One found that women on the Pill had nearly ten times the risk of dying from pulmonary embolism—when a blood clot reaches the heart—than women who weren't on it.

Along with the Pill's contraceptive effect on women's fertility is its impact, quite logically, on women's sexual experience. Scientists have recently discovered that a chemical produced by the Pill to stop ovulation continues to suppress testosterone levels—central to sexual desire in men and women—for up to a year after women stop taking it. This seven-year study showed women on the Pill had four times the level of sex hormone-binding globulin, which stops testosterone from circulating in the body, compared to those who had never taken it. Twelve months after they stopped using the Pill these women still had twice as much of this chemical in their bodies.

There were enormous problems with the higher dose Pills available up to 1975.

As widespread use of the Pill crosses generations we see the signs of specific side-effects and general depletion of wellbeing accumulate. Our rising infertility epidemic is one such area to which use of the Pill has contributed. In Australia one in six couples currently trying to conceive are experiencing problems—twice as many as there were in the 1970s. We also note the huge rise in childhood allergies, diabetes and learning and behaviour problems such as attention deficit disorder and attention deficit hyperactivity disorder.

Of great concern are the remote, hidden and ever-mounting changes within the human race, resulting from the accumulative effect of hormonal manipulation on succeeding generations. The use of the Pill must be regarded as one of the most serious and influential causes of iatrogenic disease [disease caused by a doctor].

DR DAVID LILLEY, MEDICAL PRACTITIONER AND HOMEOPATH

Manufacturers hope to allay our fears by using language suggesting safety, naturalness and benefits of the Pill—like 'mini-Pill', 'new generation' and 'low dose'. While current contraceptive pills are certainly lower in dose than those available in the 1960s and 1970s they're still many times higher than our natural hormone levels.[4] Menstrual suppression, we're also told, is more 'natural' than regular cycling and will save us from some disease states like ovarian cancer.

The Pill is big business

If you're using the Pill you'll know it can cost you anything from one hundred to several hundred dollars per year, on top of doctors' fees. Globally hormonal contraception is a multi-billion dollar industry with sales of $US1.7 billion every year in the United States alone.[5] So, as with other products, we need to be sophisticated consumers and distinguish commercials from real information. Drug advertisements aim to look like concern for our health and lifestyle, offering us 'helpful' solutions. And, as with all advertising, we can be susceptible to a good sales pitch.

A recent study for the Inspector General's Office of the US Department of Health and Human Services disclosed that more than seven out of ten advertisements for the Pill in medical publications were 'misleading or unbalanced'—making contraceptives the most 'deceptively advertised' category of prescription drug, with antibiotics in second place.[6]

Bottom drawer syndrome

A strategy well known in research circles is 'bottom drawer syndrome' where unfavourable research results are left unpublished and hopefully forgotten. There are other filtering mechanisms which also influence what research is done and what research becomes public.

The drug company Wyeth, which manufactures contraceptive Pills containing third-generation desogestrel, commissioned a study that found these Pills *significantly* increased the risk of venous thromboembolism, or blood clots. They decided not to publish the study. In 1999 independent researchers published similar findings about these Pills. Under pressure, Wyeth eventually published their results.

When we hear research findings quoted we need to ask: who is paying for this research? Who is designing the research questions and procedures? Who decides whether the research is published or not? And, who produces the information *we* receive about contraception?

A potent cocktail

The Pill, and other hormonal contraception, delivers approximately four times the corresponding oestrogen and progesterone naturally occurring at their peak in a normal menstrual cycle. These forms of contraception need to alter our fertility and hormonal balance *significantly* in order to work.

> Ingredients of Pill formulations include: ethinyl oestradiol, mestranol, levonorgestrel, norethisterone, desogestrel, gestodene, cyproterone acetate and drospirenone to name a few. These are all potent synthetic steroids.

If you're considering taking the Pill you may find it interesting to know how powerful our naturally produced hormones are and how little is needed for healthy human functioning. Hormones are generally measured in *parts per trillion*. So, in order to collect a teaspoon of oestradiol—our most prolific natural oestrogen—we'd need to distil the blood of 250 000 women of childbearing age. This gives you an idea of how exquisite and finely balanced our hormones are, and the benefit of gentle methods for balancing them when necessary, rather than effectively smashing our body's warning lights with synthetic hormones.

The Pill masks signs of reproductive health or imbalance. This creates more of a challenge for the practitioner to really be able to detect and treat any underlying imbalance in women on the Pill.

DR CLAUDIA WELCH

Some types of Pill are known as Combined Oral Contraception, which means they contain synthetic oestrogen and progesterone. These contain either the same oestrogen and progesterone dose throughout the cycle or variable quantities creating two or three phases during a cycle. Others are Progesterone-Only Pills and are often called the mini-Pill. By having no oestrogen these don't generally inhibit ovulation, although some with higher doses will.

Besides pills there are several other means of using hormonal contraception. Contraceptive injections are a way of delivering synthetic progesterone without having to remember to take a pill every day. These are injected directly into the muscle of your upper arm or buttock every four or twelve weeks. The most common brand name is Depo-Provera™. Implants are another way and are small rods inserted under the skin of your inside upper arm. They work by continuous release of synthetic progesterone into your bloodstream over three years. Norplant™ was an early, and now discredited, implant of six rods. Implanon™ is now the most widely known and is a single rod.

Intrauterine devices which slowly release synthetic progesterone are recent incarnations of earlier IUDs and are known as LNG-IUD or IUS. These are small flexible devices, made of metal and/or plastic, which are inserted into your uterus for five or more years. A widely available LNG-IUD is Mirena™.

Vaginal rings are another option. To use one you insert it high into your vagina on day one of your cycle where it stays for three weeks, then it's removed to allow for a withdrawal bleed. After seven days a new ring is inserted. Vaginal rings release synthetic oestrogen and progesterone. Nuva Ring™ is a brand of vaginal ring.

Transdermal patches are another way of delivering synthetic oestrogen and progesterone, in this case through your skin via a band-aid-like square stuck onto the skin of your buttock, upper outer arm, belly or upper torso, but not your breasts. A new patch is applied weekly for three weeks before a patch-free week allows for a withdrawal bleed.[7 & 8] Ortho Evra™ is the most common brand of contraceptive patch.

A Pill for every woman

Where chemical contraception is concerned we're led to believe that there are dramatically different formulations and these have different therapeutic outcomes. While there *are* some small statistical differences, these are greatly exaggerated when promoting various brands to doctors.

In the United States and New Zealand, where the advertising of prescription drugs to the public is legal, the path to the consumer is more direct than in countries like Australia and the United Kingdom, where it isn't. Whether their message is for us or comes via our doctor, pharmaceutical companies naturally want to show all the possible benefits of their Pill formulations in the best light they can to sell more product for a greater variety of conditions—this is simply normal business practice.

So, when considering the Pill you may like to weigh up the prolific messages of a cashed-up multinational drug industry doing brisk business against the simple voice of common sense. According to Dr David Lilley, 'Fertility is a symptom of health and infertility, resulting from chemical suppression, must equate with ill-health, resulting in malfunction and ultimately disease.'[9]

CHAPTER 3

THE NEVER-ENDING PREGNANCY

Are you on the Pill and feeling bloated? Is your appetite out of control? Are you gaining weight? Are you feeling vague, bitchy, disconnected? Are you nauseous? Are your breasts tender? Or perhaps you're feeling moody, unbalanced, neurotic, just not yourself. Do you have bouts of uncontrollable crying for no reason?

A great many of the commonly experienced side-effects of the Pill are disconcertingly similar to some of the more unpleasant symptoms that can accompany pregnancy. This is not surprising, really. To be an effective contraception the Pill induces a biochemical state in the body more like pregnancy than normal fertility. It does this by stopping ovulation and making cervical mucus impenetrable and the lining of the uterus unreceptive to implantation by an embryo.

I would wake up in middle of the night feeling nauseous—like if I'd move
I'd vomit . . . then it would go away.
WENDY, 27

However, the Pill's hormonal influence doesn't stop there. When Mena Soory, an expert in gum disease, looked at women on the Pill she found they were a third more likely to have gingivitis and higher plaque levels than if they weren't taking it. This is no coincidence, because pregnant women also suffer unusually high levels of gum disease. This is due to their raised hormone levels, which aggravate and inflame gum tissue. The difference is that for pregnant women this returns to normal after giving birth. Years of taking the Pill, however, prolong this effect and can cause lasting gum damage.[1]

There's also an elevated risk of thrombosis, or blood clots, in women on the Pill and those who are pregnant. This is due to the changes in hormonal levels to maintain a pregnancy that also increases the blood's clotting capacities. Similar to gum disease there is a greater risk of thrombosis for a woman on the Pill, compared to pregnancy, when the Pill is taken for years on end.

> Hormones affect how we think and feel and how we think and feel affects our hormones.

Biochemically speaking, the Pill induces a state similar to pregnancy *so that you won't get pregnant*.

Your hormonal messengers

So how does the Pill work? The synthetic hormones in the Pill mimic your natural hormones. They alter your hormonal balance to make you temporarily infertile and to do this they act upon your endocrine system.

Your endocrine system produces a vast array of hormones that are sent from one part of your body and are received in the receptor sites of another. In this way they convey messages about what's going on in your body and trigger specific responses. Hormones help to regulate all the processes of your body, like digestion, temperature, growth, reproduction and the chemical make-up of your blood.

Since hormones were first discovered experts in the field have found out more and more about the subtle and complex dance of hormones and their effects. There is still much more to discover and understand. What is clear, however, is that we need to approach our endocrine systems with great care and respect.

Hormones affect how we think and feel, and how we think and feel affects our hormones. They fluctuate with our moods and emotions and have often been called the molecules of emotion. We know that laughter changes our hormonal responses and affects our pain threshold—people with depression have very different brain–hormone patterns than those without—and that relaxation has a different hormonal profile than does stress.

Hormones are also your body's means of connecting the external world to your internal world, sensing and responding to changes in external stimulus like temperature, safety and comfort.

Your master endocrine gland is the hypothalamus, which has been likened to the conductor of an orchestra. This gland is located deep in your brain. The hypothalamus listens for the hormonal messages coming back from your organs, glands and tissues. It then advises the pituitary gland to send messages out to the numerous glands in your body in order to maintain a dynamic hormonal balance. The hypothalamus and pituitary work around the clock to synchronise your bodily functions, to help you to survive, cope with the effects of stress, assist your digestion, regulate your sleep–wake cycle and support your fertility.

The hormones that perform these intricate orchestrations in your body do so in exquisitely small quantities as they are immensely powerful. When blood hormone levels are being tested they are usually recorded in parts per trillion, even the most prolific ones.

Many women only realise the effect the Pill has had on them when they come off it. They often report a much greater feeling of wellbeing, both physical and psychological, as well as see improvements in specific conditions.

FRANCESCA NAISH, NATUROPATH

During a normal menstrual cycle your sex hormone levels fluctuate considerably. This creates measurable changes in *most of your body functions*—including your temperature, metabolism, nutritional uptake, blood sugar levels, blood acidity, your heart rate, your urine, the size of your pupils, your pain threshold, your brain waves, your senses of sight, sound and smell, your breasts, cervical mucus secretion, the size, position and colour of your cervix and the size and colour of your vulva, sexual interest and response and your sleep and energy cycles, to name a few.

As you peruse this list you won't be surprised to learn that while the Pill induces the hormonal effect of infertility, its impact isn't limited to your ovaries, uterus and cervix. The Pill alters at least 150 bodily functions, and affects all your organs.[2]

Most women know the difference between hormonal health and imbalance. When our hormones are all over the place this can lead to an array of health problems as well as emotional distress. *And*, this can be caused by the minutest upset of your hormone levels. Given that we still know relatively little about hormones and the endocrine system it would seem to be a good idea to take great care when contemplating any artificial changes to your hormone levels.

When I was 25 I was at a major turning point in my life. I wanted to look deeply into what my life was about and get to know myself better. So, I took up meditation in a very committed way and found many things started to change quite naturally and very positively. One change was that although I'd been on the Pill since I was seventeen I found I just couldn't take it anymore.

SERENA, 35

By altering our natural hormone levels, the Pill induces in us a *different* biochemical and psychological state. This in turn interferes with the particular psychological stage of life we're in and may affect our ongoing unfoldment thereafter, no matter which model of human development we refer to.[3] While it may be difficult to prove the effect that taking the Pill has on our psychological development we can see that through its profound hormonal impact the Pill may also be interfering with the fundamental chemistry of who we are and what we can become.

CHAPTER 4

RECOGNISING SIDE-EFFECTS

Women are frequently grateful to be offered effective contraception they can simply forget about—contraception that doesn't depend on having the headspace to remember it *every day*. These may be injections, implants or hormone releasing IUDs. After such an appealing promise of convenience and freedom many women find the result is more like a nightmare gone horribly wrong. Here Carmela tells us her story:

My obstetrician recommended the implant and said it would be just like being perpetually pregnant. 'Been there, done that, so why worry?' I thought. His confidence that this was the most reliable form of contraception was quite enough for me. I already had two sons under two. I was tired and didn't want to run any risks.

Months later... with my head resting against the wall in our spare bathroom and tears running down my face, I wondered if I had any control over myself anymore. How many times had I escaped here today? I didn't know. How many times had I abused my children verbally and then fled from them, frightened that I might soon abuse them physically as well? I didn't know. All I wanted to do was lash out.

'This is not me!' I screamed in my own mind. But who else could be doing this? How is it possible to lose control to such an extent?

I thought I was insane. Days became a blur and I lived for the moments when my children were asleep, when I didn't have to go near them and risk hurting them.

In those moments of peace I recall standing in front of our bedroom mirror and repeatedly punching myself in the face as hard as I could so that the physical need to strike out would be appeased and only I would be hurt.

I fantasised about methods of escape. Slipping out in the middle of the night and disappearing into the city, nameless. One more person sleeping under a bridge. No, I could be found. Suicide seemed my only option. My children would certainly be better off with no mother than the one they had now, and my husband would eventually find a new love who would care for our children properly. Definitely the way to go.

My husband, I convinced myself, would be glad I was gone. He too would be safe. Previously, our relationship had been the kind in which true misunderstanding occurred only rarely. Now he was frightened of me. Some days, on his return from work, I would flee the house a sobbing mess leaving him to comfort the children alone. Some days all would seem fine until the children were in bed but then I would berate him with a list of small grievances magnified into threats of divorce.

On one occasion I abused him so mercilessly that I almost drove him to an act of self-harm. He had been forced to suppress his own fear and anger at my behaviour for too long.

Finally I asked my (very nervous) husband to come with me to the doctor. Something was seriously wrong. I explained that I had 'grown horns', was angry and felt out of control. I could find no other words to describe my actions, yet these words seemed to trivialise the desperation I was experiencing. I was sure that the doctor would shrug off my concerns and I would be left with nowhere to turn.

Fortunately the doctor was really kind. He asked if I was taking any medication and simply nodded when I told him I had a contraceptive device in my arm—the implant was releasing measured doses of progesterone into my system, like some contraceptive pills but without the concern of forgetting to take a pill. 'We'll take that out and you'll be fine,' was his response. We questioned the doctor repeatedly, wondering how he could be so sure that was the problem. The doctor was sure and, in his certainty, very comforting.

A follow-up appointment was made so he could remove the implant from my arm with the assistance of a nurse. A couple of days passed that were filled with hope—had we found an answer?—and even greater fear—what if it was not the answer? What then? Committal?

Finally, my husband stayed home with the boys and I cried my way to the surgery. I'll never forget the nurse's comment when I told her how long I had had the implant. She very calmly remarked, 'Oh, and you haven't killed anyone yet?'

'What?'

'It's the progestogen.'

The very calm manner in which she made this statement chilled me. How many other people were having this implant removed for the same reasons?

Out it came and home I went, thinking very carefully. If life went back to normal from now, I would forget the whole thing. If I continued to act like the spawn of Satan, I would have to summon up the courage to return and ask for a psychiatric assessment.

Within two days I was once more able to think clearly and hold my temper. It took longer, maybe a couple of weeks, for me to modify certain behaviours that had become habitual under the influence of the implant, but I was able to find the control to do so. I was no longer helpless. All it took was the flick of a razor blade, which, despite my worst fears, had been wielded by my doctor and not by me.

However, my intention to forget has been impossible to fulfil.

So many of us are prescribed drugs of various kinds. We have a prescription filled and glance cursorily over the accompanying information sheet, which, of course, we know is very important. If we see a statement along the lines of 'May cause mood swings' or 'May cause depression', we think, Not me, I'm in control and that won't happen to me. These statements and warnings are provided for valid reasons and I know I should have paid closer attention. I can only thank my doctor for seeing the problem and the solution so very quickly. It had taken months of fearing for my children's lives to get me moving.

Today I am myself again. I feel defeated by the size of the ironing pile but, let's face it, ironing doesn't really matter. I get upset when the boys turn up their noses at the superb meal I have spent the last hour and a half preparing. Their favourite foods at the moment are cheese, sausages, dried pears and sultanas so I really should know better. I have two very gifted performers who occasionally treat me to world-class synchronised tantrums. I have learned that a raised eyebrow and banishment to the 'couch' does the trick and saves me the energy of getting involved. Should they manage to suck me into the excitement, I head for my own 'couch' for thinking time.

I am myself again and my husband is very grateful.

Side-effects from the Pill, implants and other hormonal contraception are real, common and can be devastating. These aren't always recognised as resulting from the drug as quickly as in Carmela's case. Some develop slowly as an accumulation of effects. Some may make existing health problems worse. Some may be explained away as having other causes. Some are just tolerated. If you're on the Pill or using other hormonal contraception, or considering it, be aware of the potential side-effects and monitor your health very carefully. Take the time to learn about other methods so that you have real options and alternatives.

In packets of the Pill you'll find warnings and information about possible side-effects. With other forms of hormonal contraception you'll be given information to read. Read it thoroughly. The manufacturers of these products are obliged by law to include lists of known side-effects. Do, however, be aware that they also take great care to word information leaflets in such a way as to suggest these side-effects are rare, and can happen to women who don't take the Pill as well. So, who can really say why *you* get depressed or put on weight after starting the Pill? For drug companies it's simply good business for women to doubt that the Pill is the cause of their distress.

> For drug companies it's simply good business for women to doubt that the Pill is the cause of their distress.

Most women who have ever been on the Pill have been aware of side-effects to a greater or lesser degree. That's why Pill-use peaks in women in their early to mid-twenties, and tapers off as they find other means to regulate their fertility.

Many girls and women using hormonal contraception will have several side-effects at the same time. Most commonly these include mood swings, depression, appetite changes, weight gain and loss of sex drive. Unlike Carmela's doctor, many don't recognise the effects so promptly and women are often encouraged to keep taking the Pill, despite the side-effects, in the expectation that things will settle down, or that the Pill isn't the cause. As far as your body and contraception are concerned, we encourage you to listen closely and take note. Take the time to observe and trust your own perceptions and reactions. This will help you to know what effect the drug does or does not have on *your* body.

> All drugs have side-effects; the big question is, are the side-effects worth the benefits?

Some side-effects are a direct result of introducing synthetic chemicals into your body which then mimic but are not identical to the hormones you naturally

An analysis of studies into the Pill found the side-effects of combined oral contraceptives included depression, nausea, vomiting, headaches, urinary and lower genital tract infections.

produce. These synthetic hormones are approximately four times stronger than your natural hormone levels. While the influence of a mechanical contraceptive procedure or device is more likely to be limited to a specific area of your body, chemicals are distributed throughout your body via your bloodstream and affect all organs and processes. *All* the drugs we take have side-effects—the big question we all struggle with is whether the side-effects are worth the benefits.

Some women have such obvious and severe side-effects when they take the Pill they soon stop. Others may have some symptoms but put up with them because they need contraception and for the sake of their relationship. Others have no obvious symptoms, and continue to take the Pill year after year, decade after decade.

Some may be girls too young to know themselves and their bodies well enough to understand how they would normally feel and what effect the drug is having on them. As they mature, and have only known themselves as a woman on the Pill, health and emotional imbalances may be seen as normal, even though unpleasant.

All these women will have side-effects whether they or their doctors attribute their health issues to the Pill or not. And, what's more, these effects aren't limited to ourselves.

The men in our lives are also affected. When we consider the side-effects of the Pill we may think the burden is ours alone, but depression, loss of libido and chronic health problems can seriously impact and concern our partners as well.

I really noticed a difference in my girlfriend when she started taking the Pill. She became a lot more emotional and just not as clear somehow.

DAVID, 26

Often the risks and side-effects of the Pill are weighed against the health risks and side-effects of pregnancy. This would be valid if there were no other way to avoid an unplanned conception, but there are many. And, the good news is that there are lots of alternatives which don't interfere with your biochemistry. Later we'll look at different approaches to contraception, and how to find out what's most suitable, and will work best, for you.

CHAPTER 5

FEELING DEPRESSED?

According to the World Health Organization, one in four women experience clinical depression in their lifetime as compared with one in six men. While not a happy statistic on any level, depression in men and women is also the fourth leading contributor to the global burden of disease. Experts suggest that by 2020 it will become the *second* leading contributor.[1]

Professor Jayashri Kulkani, a psychiatrist, says that, 'Depression is one of the most prevalent and debilitating illnesses affecting the female population today.' In her research into the effects of the Pill on mood Professor Kulkani found that women taking the Pill were *almost twice* as likely to be depressed compared to those not on the Pill. The women in the study were over eighteen, none were pregnant or breastfeeding, they had no clinical history of depression and none had been on anti-depressants in the previous twelve months.[2 & 3]

I was never diagnosed as depressed but I was often suicidal, withdrawn, crying, angry and aggressive.
MADELINE, 35

A government body set up to gather and provide information about adverse psychiatric reactions to drugs has hundreds of case studies of women who said they suffered depression, mood swings and self-harm while on one leading oral contraceptive, which is also used as a hormone treatment for acne and excessive hair growth.[4]

Madeline was on the Pill for contraception and irregular cycles for fifteen years, from age eighteen. 'Overall I believe the Pill contributed to my mood swings,' she confessed. 'I was never diagnosed as depressed but I was often suicidal, withdrawn, crying, angry and aggressive.' And Anna found that while she was on the Pill, 'Emotional flare-ups and depression placed a lot of stress on my relationship. My husband was very supportive, but couldn't really understand why I would just cry and have periods of anger and depression.'

Health profession journals regularly publish information about the negative effects women have while on the Pill. In these articles oral contraceptive use has been associated with increased rates of depression, divorce, tranquilliser use, sexual dysfunction and suicide. Several studies have shown that women taking the Pill, or other hormonal contraception, were also found to have higher rates of anxiety, fatigue, neurotic symptoms, compulsion, anger and negative menstrual effects.[5]

A review of multiple studies into the Pill found the side-effects of combined oral contraceptives included depression, nausea, vomiting, headaches, urinary and lower genital tract infections.[6] And in a large ongoing study of 23 000 oral contraception users over a third of the women on the Pill stopped taking it *because of depression*.[7] Furthermore, a study of 139 girls whose average age was sixteen and who were on the Pill for contraceptive and therapeutic reasons, revealed that their most common side-effects were weight gain, an increase in their breast size, fatigue and *depression*.[8] Given the sheer weight of research and women's experiences connecting the Pill to depression, we have to wonder: why don't we have much stronger checks and balances around prescribing girls and women the Pill?

In Chapter 11 when we consider the complex mix of the Pill's disruption of our normal ability to process nutrients, we can see why so many women experience these distressing symptoms. In particular absorption is disrupted in Vitamins B1, B2, B6 and B12 leading to deficiency, and the zinc/copper balance is disturbed—all of which can lead to depression and mood disorders.

In the next chapter we'll look in detail at research that found a hormone-binding globulin that is seven times higher in women on the Pill and four times higher in women *who have ever taken it*, compared to those who haven't. This globulin binds with testosterone and takes it out of circulation. Studies have shown that when there's a change, up or down, to normal testosterone levels in women, it can cause depression. Oral contraception clearly causes a decline in women's testosterone levels resulting in depression and mood disorders for many women.[9]

When I was on the Pill I loved the spontaneity [of sexual expression] but the moods were scary stuff.

IRENA, 26

Given the vast number of women on the Pill and the proportion of those who experience depression, mood swings and other psychological and emotional disturbances from the drug, we can see that there's a *significant* proportion of the population who are both on the Pill and depressed because of it. It's sobering to realise that use of the Pill adds considerably to the total number of women suffering depression in our community and globally. Many of these remain on the Pill for years despite their symptoms, either because neither they nor their doctor have connected the depression to the drug, or because they don't feel they have any alternative. For any individual this is painful and life-draining. Society-wide it's an unnecessary tragedy and may amount to gross neglect.

For those fortunate women whose doctors quickly see the connection, like Carmela, their suffering can be short-lived. For many others like Kim, the suffering goes on year after year. As women we need to know the Pill can have a profound impact on our choices, our relationships and family life, our career, our self-esteem and our health. Too often women struggle with many issues that the Pill creates assuming it's all 'them'. For the many women who start taking the Pill as teenagers by the time they're adults they only know themselves on the Pill. It's often only years later when they go off the Pill that they're able to connect the dots and see the symptoms that it caused.

> If you are on the Pill, or any of its relatives, and any of these women's stories sound familiar, please consider that it may be the synthetic hormones you're taking that are causing your distress.

After six months on the Pill I had nausea for the first three or four hours every day, was depressed and just wanted to cry all the time. My doctor thought this was because I was studying psychology. I decided to stop taking the Pill and felt much better.

TONI, 28

Ella was on the Pill for nineteen years. During this time her mood swings were severe. 'Some doctors were quite sympathetic,' Ella recalls, 'others said the moods were completely unrelated to the Pill.' Irena had the same side-effects to battle. She was on the Pill from age sixteen to 33, and had terrible mood swings and premenstrual symptoms. 'I was teary, angry and very emotional. The main positive was the availability of sexual expression without condoms or diaphragms,' she admits. 'I loved the spontaneity. But the moods were scary stuff. I got my repeat scripts over the phone without any review.'

If you are on the Pill, or any of its relatives, and any of these women's stories sound familiar, please consider that it may be the synthetic hormones you're taking that are causing your distress. Whether you're taking the Pill for menstrual problems, skin problems, or for contraception, consider switching to one of the very good alternatives available to you for each of these purposes.

I was amazed. I woke in the morning feeling refreshed, awake and alive. I had a feeling of happiness and an absence from depression that I was very unfamiliar with!

KIM, 37

CHAPTER 6

LOW LIBIDO —IS *THAT* HOW IT WORKS?

The Pill can look like a real boon to your relationship. It promises worry-free sex and control over messy periods so that they don't interrupt your sex life. Initially a woman may feel freer, and certainly for men, who don't have the emotional and physical side-effects, the Pill seems to offer nothing but pluses.

Feeling totally confident about their contraception can be a powerful aphrodisiac in itself for many women. For Susie, 'Being able to have unprotected sex with my partner was great. I felt closer to him.' And Helena enjoyed having 'No threat of babies. We could have sex anytime with no restrictions.'

While effective contraception is of course the primary reason women go on the Pill, and faith in their contraception does help a woman relax and enjoy her sex life, she may also be damaging her capacity for deep sexual pleasure.

The Pill flattens out natural oestradiol highs and suppresses free testosterone, potentially delivering a double libido blow.

PROFESSOR LORRAINE DENNERSTEIN

When we consider the side-effects that many women experience on the Pill—like mood swings, depression, weight gain, headaches or migraine—we find that these impact a woman's self-esteem and in turn her capacity to establish or maintain a healthy sexual relationship.

Peter is a 23-year-old computer technician and has noticed that his girlfriends on the Pill seemed to be sick a lot: 'They have a general malaise and fatigue while women off the Pill seem freer.' His current girlfriend is not using the Pill and 'has much more energy and sexual drive than previous girlfriends who were on it.' For Peter this is a much better state of affairs and he's more than happy to share responsibility for contraception.

At first taking the Pill was positive because sex was free from worry, but after a while, when the side-effects kicked in, I began to feel resentful that I was risking my health and blamed my partner. Our relationship became more distant and our sexual relationship lost its intimacy and honesty, especially after my moods became erratic.

LALLI, 32

Unfortunately even the Pill's reputation for effectiveness is not matched by the facts—of the 60 million women who are on the Pill in the United States and Europe *two million a year* have an unplanned pregnancy. When a woman has an unwanted pregnancy on the Pill, or learns of the extent of the risk, the aphrodisiac effect can quickly evaporate.

The chemical fallout

Many women who take the Pill and whose libido plummets along with their fertility have wondered, 'Is *that* how it works?'. If we take a medication that alters the natural cycle of our primary reproductive hormones, perhaps we should *expect* this to impact our sexuality as well.

Professor Lorraine Dennerstein speaking on television in 2004 noted that it's strange that we have pharmaceutical companies spending millions of dollars trying to develop a pill that improves women's sexual interest or arousal, while at the same time we liberally distribute the oral contraceptive Pill, which suppresses women's sexual function—with about one-third of women on the Pill experiencing adverse effects on their sexuality from it.

> Common side-effects of the Pill—like mood swings, depression, weight gain, headaches or migraine—impact a woman's self-esteem and wellbeing and in turn her capacity to establish or maintain a healthy sexual relationship.

She added, 'Research has found that during the normal menstrual cycle oestradiol (our primary oestrogen) rises and falls, peaking around ovulation. When this peaks so does sexual desire. This is very clever from an evolutionary point of view as it turns out that the six days in which women have a peak level of sexual desire are the same six days when we're potentially fertile. The Pill flattens out the natural oestradiol highs and suppresses testosterone, delivering a double libido blow.'[1]

I know that while I was on the Pill my libido wasn't very high. I was less sensitive and had dryness and tension during sex.
NINA, 27

Perhaps the most definitive research about the effects of the Pill on libido was carried out by Dr Irwin Goldstein and Dr Claudia Panzer. They found that taking the Pill for as little as six months could potentially destroy a woman's sex drive forever. The Pill dramatically reduces the levels of testosterone, which is vital to both female and male libido, and simply stopping taking the Pill doesn't necessarily reverse this effect.

Doctors Goldstein and Panzer studied 125 women: 62 were on the Pill, 40 had taken it in the past and 23 had never taken it. Those on it and those who had taken it in the past had been on it for at least six months. The women were tested every three months for a year, measuring their levels of sex hormone-binding globulin, a protein which binds with testosterone and takes it out of circulation. They found that levels of this hormone-binding globulin were *seven times higher* in Pill users than in those who had never taken it. Among those who had taken it in the past but not currently, levels were still three to four times higher—effectively removing testosterone and crippling libido indefinitely.

Other research has found the effects of the Pill on sexual enjoyment and libido include diminished or complete loss of sexual interest and arousal, muted or non-existent orgasms, decreased frequency of sexual intercourse and significantly more sexual pain reported by women taking the Pill compared with those who had never taken it.[2] Similarly the Pill can lead to sore and cystic breasts, secretions from the breast, vaginal discharges and a much greater tendency for vaginal thrush, vaginal dryness, period pain, spotting and breakthrough bleeding, cervical erosions, systemic candida infection, a greater tendency for genital warts and chlamydial infection, all of which can affect libido and sexual pleasure.

> *When the Pill is handed out like candy I don't think doctors always tell*
> *women about potential side-effects . . . women should know it can*
> *affect their sex lives.*
> **DR CLAUDIA PANZER**

Of course a great many factors can affect our sexual desire and the ebb and flow of our sexuality can seem, at times, an impenetrable mystery. Nonetheless the research on the Pill and libido offers us some very clear indicators. Although not all women on the Pill will experience the change in their sex hormone-binding globulin levels or their hormonal cycle as diminished libido it is clear that many will.

I've seen this [loss of libido] for years in many patients on the Pill, and was very happy to learn of this new research.

DR CHRISTIANE NORTHRUP

The animal in us

A fascinating study by primatologist Ron Nadler shows a direct connection between hormones and lust, and that for females the relationship itself is a potent part of sexual attraction.

Male orang-utans are basically always ready for sexual activity. Nadler wanted to see what would happen if he gave the female orang-utans the power to choose when *they* wanted to have sex. He put males and females in side-by-side cages with a door between them that the females could pass through but were too small for the males. Most of the time the females were content to simply admire the males through the bars, using the door only when they were ovulating.

Next Nadler studied groups of chimpanzees, in which the larger, more aggressive males also dominated, and he separated the males and females similarly. The male could only reach the female if *she* pushed a lever to open the connecting door—the door lever was only on her side.

There were nine pairs of chimpanzees in the study, and Nadler looked at their behaviour when the females were both on and off the Pill. When the females were on the Pill the door stayed shut more often and sexual relations declined steadily for seven of the pairs. With one of the remaining pairs, who apparently had a terrific relationship, both sexually and companionably, the oral contraceptive made no real difference at all—they threw open the door and mated with undiminished enthusiasm. With the remaining pair the male had aggressively intimidated the female and mating habits were also basically undisturbed. In other words, when the female chimpanzees operated the door, the frequency of sex diminished *unless* there was a strong relationship (of either compatibility or male domination) to override the hormonal effects.[3]

I have a low sex drive. I don't know if this is Pill related or not as I have never been off the Pill. This makes it hard for my husband as he wants sex more than I do.

DIANA, 34

Just friends

A recent study found that women on the Pill see the world more platonically. Female medical students who were both on and off the Pill were showed images of naked men and women. Those on the Pill were far less likely to imagine sexual scenarios as they viewed these pictures, seeing them more as neutral compositions of muscle, bone and skin, than those not on the Pill. They were also less likely to be charmed by pictures of babies—hinting at the Pill's influence on reproductive interest.[4]

If you're struggling to attract a boyfriend here's another factor to consider. Certain volatile fatty acids—wonderfully named 'copulins'—are secreted in the vagina and stimulate male sexual interest and behaviour. Women on the Pill, however, *don't secrete copulins*.[5] We can only guess at how many other ways the Pill may be impacting our hormonal and sexual balance. How many men would be willing for their sexual appetite or attractiveness to be similarly eroded?

Many women express how differently they feel after coming off the Pill. Vivien found 'The Pill's effect on my relationship was not good—total disinterest in sex and recurring thrush caused major problems between us. Once I was off the Pill I was much better in myself, although the thrush took two years to get rid of.' Anna says, 'No more emotional outbursts, I feel great! My sex drive has increased heaps!' and Melinda adds, 'How do I feel coming off the Pill? FREE!! Orgasmic, sensual, sexual, lusty, confident, wonderful!'

Need we say more?

CHAPTER 7

MOOD SWINGS, WEIGHT GAIN, BRITTLE BONES AND MIGRAINES

Your liver is your largest internal organ and has a wider range of functions than any other organ in your body. Among other things it processes nutrients and detoxifies your blood. Taking the Pill places considerable strain on your liver. That's because it's your liver's job to break down the synthetic hormones before they're distributed to the rest of your body. As your gall bladder works closely with your liver the effect of the extra load of the Pill on your body is reflected in a greater risk of gallstone disease[1] as well as liver cancer.[2]

> It's oral contraception that particularly exposes the liver to a toxic load.

Nausea, crankiness and moodiness, as well as feeling depleted, tired and rundown, can in part be traced to this added strain that processing the Pill places on your liver. The synthetic oestrogens in all but the mini-Pill can cause the liver to produce higher levels of blood clotting substances than it otherwise would, leading to a greater risk of blood clots in women on the Pill.[3]

Of the various forms of chemical contraception it's oral contraception that *particularly* exposes the liver to this toxic load. As contraceptive implants, injections, hormone impregnated IUDs, vaginal rings and patches all deliver hormones directly to your bloodstream rather than through your stomach, gut and liver, these are preferred by some doctors who are concerned about their patient's vulnerable livers. Best not get too excited about this, though, as these other forms of contraception are still delivering strong doses of synthetic hormones to your body so that your liver, while not an initial recipient, will eventually get its share.

> *I was suffering overall ADR (ain't doin' right) on the Pill—depressed, lethargic and cranky. I was fed up and looking for a solution.*
> **JACINTA, 23**

Jane Lyttleton, a practitioner of Traditional Chinese Medicine (TCM), tells us that 'the Pill interferes with normal Liver qi [energetic flow] function in the body leading to Liver stagnation in many women'. When a woman decides to stop taking the Pill her TCM treatment includes 'liver support to rid her body of excess hormones'.[4] Paulette notices that 'I get sick often when I'm on the Pill—throat and chest infections and colds—and I'm tired all the time'. For some women just coming off the Pill can be a great boost to their sense of wellbeing. Kim found that, 'When I came off the Pill I felt energetic and really positive. People asked me what drug was making me so happy!'

> For women using Depo-Provera™ predictable weight gain in the first year is 2.5 kilograms and after two years it's 3.7 kilograms.

Not fat and happy

Meena had always been happy with her weight before having a contraceptive implant inserted into her upper arm. Even though her eating and routine didn't change, she gained fifteen kilograms in just six months. Although she was glad to have reliable contraception, Meena began to feel upset and self-conscious about her weight and this quickly had repercussions on her relationship. She wished the likelihood of weight gain had been explained to her: 'I wouldn't have chosen the implant if I'd had any idea this would happen,' she admits. Now, some years after having the implant removed, Meena is still working to regain something close to her previous weight.

Weight gain is one of the *most* common side-effects of the Pill. Not only can this affect our body image, self-esteem and general health, but it may also cascade into a whole string of health problems, including eating disorders, overweight, obesity and diabetes. Occasionally a woman loses weight on the Pill; however, this is usually the case for women who least want it.

The hormonal and nutritional disturbance of the Pill can impact appetite as well as mood, and may be a contributing factor for some girls and young women who develop eating disorders. When Andrea was fifteen she went on the Pill. She remembers that 'I was hungry all the time and had dark moods I couldn't manage,' and admits, 'I developed a binge and purge habit to cope, and it took me some years to find my own way through the emotional mess. It was only much later that I realised the Pill had played a critical role.'

Predictable weight gain

For women using Depo-Provera™ *predictable weight gain* in the first year of use is 2.5 kilograms. Then after two years it's 3.7 kilograms. After four years this rises to 6.3 kilograms. If you are considering using this form of contraception you may also want to think about whether or not you want to gain weight.

Ironically if you are overweight or obese chemical contraception will be less effective for you. A recent study found that women on the Pill who weighed 70 kilos or more were 60 per cent more likely to have an unplanned pregnancy. Seventy kilos isn't much more than an average woman's weight—which is 66 kilos in Australia—so you don't have to be that much heavier to be at a higher risk of pregnancy even though you're on the Pill.[5]

I felt horrible on the Pill. I was gaining weight and felt sluggish and domesticated, like a farm animal.

LISA, 43

Although Rhiannon was on the Pill she got pregnant. After much discussion with her boyfriend she decided to have an abortion. Her doctor then advised that Depo-Provera™ injections would offer her better contraception. She bled constantly for the first three months until she was given the Pill to take as well. From the first time she had the injection Rhiannon found she changed from being a happy, down to earth, outgoing woman to being submissive, shy and insecure. She developed panic attacks, depression and chronic fatigue, and lost half the thickness of the hair on her head.

Before Depo-Provera™ Rhiannon had successfully lost 20 kilos of excess weight. She was proud of herself and felt in control. When she had the injection she found her weight just wouldn't budge even though she was on the same nutrition and exercise program. After three Depo-Provera™

> A recent study of women aged eighteen to 39 on the Pill who weighed 70 kilos or more found that they were 60 per cent more likely to have their birth control pills fail than women who weighed less.

shots she stopped. She is now pre-diabetic and distressed to discover that using the Pill, and contraceptive injections, increased her risk of diabetes.[6]

All forms of hormonal contraception—even the mini-Pill—have been shown to cause weight gain and increase your tendency to deposit cellulite.[7] They do this through suppressing thyroid function, inducing testosterone deficiency and insulin resistance. The latter increases the risk of cardiovascular disease, diabetes and polycystic ovarian syndrome.[8] It may be worth remembering that synthetic oestrogens are fed to beef cattle to *make* them gain weight.

Polycystic ovarian syndrome

It's estimated that between one in ten and one in twenty women of child-bearing age have polycystic ovarian syndrome. The classic symptoms of this are weight gain, failure to ovulate, infrequent periods, infertility, facial hair, acne, loss of hair from the head, reduced libido, exhaustion, reduced mental alertness, depression, anxiety and a predisposition to diabetes.

Recent research found the Pill to be the most commonly prescribed therapy for managing polycystic ovarian symptoms. However, a growing number of doctors are concerned that the Pill only increases the risk of diabetes in polycystic patients and exacerbates other symptoms. Many are turning to more natural and lifestyle based therapy programs.

Francesca Naish, a naturopath and reproductive health expert, treats many women with polycystic ovarian syndrome. She says that while not all women with this condition have insulin resistance, a high proportion do. For them taking the Pill covers up symptoms and doesn't deal with the underlying cause, which is a risk factor for diabetes. Francesca finds that while the specific hormonal imbalance of polycystic ovarian syndrome varies from woman to woman, many find that their condition is successfully controlled or brought into remission with natural therapies.

Down to the brittle bones

Contrary to what we believed about hormone replacement therapy and expected from the Pill—a protective strengthening of our bones—researchers have found that the oral contraceptive pill, as well as the injectable contraception Depo-Provera™, actually causes significant *loss* of bone mineral density and that this may not be completely reversible when a woman stops taking the Pill.[9 & 10]

A large study that investigated fractures among 46 000 women who had ever used the Pill found that the incidence of fracture was *significantly higher* than for women who had never used it.[11 & 12] Clearly the Pill is not going to help us maintain strong bones.

Women are often willing to trade pretty lousy side-effects for the security that they won't get pregnant.
DR CLAUDIA WELCH

In late 2004 the US Food and Drug Administration and Pfizer—the pharmaceutical company which produces Depo-Provera™—notified healthcare professionals of revisions to the safety labelling of Depo-Provera™ to include 'black label' warnings of significant bone mineral density loss associated with its use, a loss that increases the longer it's used and may not be completely reversible. The warning also says that a woman should use Depo-Provera™ for no more than two years, and only if other methods of contraception have proved inadequate. Particular caution is advised in early adulthood and adolescence—the time of life *the majority* of women begin to use chemical contraception.

Some evidence exists that increasing dietary calcium—by having a medium or high dairy diet of 1000 to 1300 milligrams of calcium a day—may prevent spine and hip bone density loss for young women using the Pill.[13] We need to remember, however, that a high dairy diet may present other problems for some women and needs to be considered alongside overall nutritional needs and sensitivities.

What! Another headache?

Kate went on the Pill at eighteen to treat her irregular and painful periods. Unfortunately it didn't make a difference to her monthly pain but she stayed on it for contraceptive purposes. While on the Pill she started having migraines during the week before each period as well as mood swings, crying jags and feeling tired and light-headed. Kate asked her doctor, 'Could the migraines be caused by the Pill?' He didn't think so. Finally when she was 25 Kate took herself off the Pill and she hasn't had a single migraine since.

A recent large study found that women who take oral contraceptives containing synthetic oestrogen have increased chances of suffering from both migraine and non-migraine headaches. Migraines were found to be 40 per cent more common and non-migraine headaches 20 per cent more common among Pill users compared to women not taking the Pill. The relative quantity of oestrogen didn't seem to make any difference. Researchers thought this was because even the lowest dose of synthetic oestrogen is still four times a woman's natural level. The migraine and non-migraine headaches mainly occurred during the placebo-pill days—triggered by the sharp drop in oestrogen levels. Effectively the headaches were monthly drug-withdrawal symptoms.[14]

For other women who already experience migraines taking the Pill can seriously exacerbate these problems, as in the case of Elaine, who had suffered from migraines, dizziness and fainting spells since around the time of her first period when she was eleven years old. When she was sixteen Elaine went on the Pill and continued to have migraines, believing they were something she had to live with. At 21 she

> The migraine and non-migraine headaches mainly occurred during the placebo-pill days—effectively the headaches were monthly withdrawal symptoms.

consulted a gynaecologist who tried her on another brand of Pill to see if it would make a difference to the migraines—it didn't. He asked her if she was comfortable having migraines and being on the Pill. Not being aware of the risks she was taking she said yes, meaning she could cope with the migraines as she was used to them.

> Women who take oral contraceptives containing synthetic oestrogen have increased chances of suffering from both migraine and non-migraine headaches.

Then, when she was 25, Elaine suffered a mild stroke during the visual disturbance before a migraine. It took four days to get a doctor or hospital to take her seriously *because she was so young* and no-one wanted to waste funds on a CT scan. In that time she permanently lost a quarter of her eyesight. Tests then revealed that Elaine had probably had an earlier stroke or two.

While the Pill was not the underlying cause of her migraines, Elaine having had them before she took it, the Pill is known to dangerously exacerbate these symptoms, and is likely to have tipped the balance towards the strokes that she had.

If you're on the Pill or other hormonal contraception, read the fine print on the product leaflet carefully. If you start having headaches or migraines, or your headaches increase in frequency, get them checked out, and seriously consider other contraception. Going on the Pill if you already have migraines, or staying on it when they start, is simply too dangerous.

CHAPTER 8

DYING NOT TO GET PREGNANT

While lethal side-effects of the Pill are rare, deaths that are *directly attributable* to the Pill do happen, and are those you most want to do without! The most common of these are cardiovascular diseases—blood clots, strokes and heart attacks—and cancer.

By 1975, in the United States, the Pill was responsible for almost the same number of deaths as those caused by pregnancy and childbirth.[1]

When the Pill is *dangerous*

It is not advisable to take the Pill if you have or have had any of the following conditions as it may bring on or exacerbate your symptoms. Avoidance or special care should also be taken if you have any family history of these: abnormal vaginal bleeding, blood clot formation, breast nodules or fibrocystic disease of the breast, Chrohn's disease, depression, diabetes, diseases triggered by pregnancy (like jaundice, herpes and chloasma), endometriosis, epilepsy, fibroid tumours of the uterus, gall bladder disease, heart or circulatory disease or stroke, high blood pressure, high cholesterol and triglycerides, kidney or liver disease, HIV disease, inflammatory bowel disease, kidney or liver disease, known or suspected breast or uterine cancer, large, swollen and tender varicose veins, liver tumours, disorders or damage, malabsorption syndrome, migraine or recurrent headaches, multiple sclerosis, obesity, periods that are too frequent or no periods at all, recurrent or active hepatitis, sickle-cell anaemia, trophoblastic disease, tuberculosis and valvular heart disease.

The Pill is also not advised for girls or women who are pregnant, suspect they may be pregnant or intend to conceive, are breastfeeding or scheduled for surgery, adolescents who have been menstruating for less than two years or for women who are over 35 years of age. And, it's also best avoided with cigarette smoking, drinking alcohol[2] and long-haul flights as these increase the risk of blood clots and other side-effects from the Pill.

> *Women on the Pill are more likely to be affected by alcohol and for a longer period of time than women who are not on the Pill and they should not mix these drugs.*
> **DR HOWARD SHAPIRO**

Similarly you shouldn't mix the Pill with drugs that induce liver enzymes, oral anticoagulant drugs, certain antibiotics, antihistamines, insulin, tranquillisers, sedatives and antidepressants, drugs for seizure disorders, steroids, St John's Wort or any hormonally active herbs.

Blood clots (also known as thrombosis, thromboembolism, venous thrombosis and pulmonary embolism)

Belinda was 24 when she flew from Melbourne to London for the start of what was meant to be her long-anticipated overseas adventure. Within 48 hours of her arrival in England Belinda tragically died from pulmonary embolism—a blood clot that had reached her heart. Her dramatic death served to finally make public the link between deep vein thrombosis and long-haul flights. That she was also on the Pill was noted and although the link between the Pill and thrombosis was known, it simply wasn't the big-news story that reporters were after at the time.

Despite efforts by pharmaceutical companies to decrease the danger of thrombosis that the Pill has posed to women with the 'third-generation' oral contraceptives that have been available since 1985, research has found that third-generation Pills actually carry a *higher risk* of blood clots.

> Research has found that third-generation Pills actually carry a higher risk of blood clots.

In 1995 when government health ministers in Britain went public with information about the increased risk of thromboembolism that third-generation contraceptive Pills posed, British women's use of the Pill dropped sharply, as did the incidence of deep vein thrombosis among oral contraceptive users.[3] While research has found that third-generation Pills have doubled the risk of thrombosis relative to second-generation Pills,[4] compared to not taking the Pill at all the risk is much higher. One study found that women who took the Pill had nearly ten times the risk of dying from pulmonary embolism than women who didn't.[5]

Tom's wife Julie died from a blood clot while taking the Pill. After her death Tom wanted to find out why his 35-year-old wife had died. He became convinced that the Pill had caused the blood clot in her ovarian vein. He took the pharmaceutical company who produced the drug to court. Although he lost the case his testimony touched the hearts of many who were there and others who later read the newspaper reports. In his grief he was able to convey that his wife was not just a statistic but a real person, the dedicated mother of their five daughters, and that her loss would be keenly felt.[6]

> Tom's wife Julie died from a blood clot while taking the Pill. She was the dedicated mother of five daughters.

As a result of substantial findings about the risk of blood clots, and with pressure from lobby groups, health authorities in many countries have insisted that information in Pill packets include warnings about thrombosis. While obeying the letter of the law careful attention is paid by manufacturers when wording these warnings so as not to alarm the consumer. A little alarm may actually be better for you. Do read warnings carefully!

Stroke and heart attack

A 25-year study of over 45 000 women found that deaths from cardio-vascular diseases like thrombosis, strokes and heart attacks were significantly increased in women on the Pill,[7] and even the lowest dose Pills have been found to cause a doubling of the risk for strokes and heart attacks.[8 & 9]

We've seen from Elaine's story (in Chapter 7) the serious consequences that occurred when her migraines were exacerbated by the Pill and she had a series of strokes.

Doctors are frequently reminded to prescribe the Pill only to women who have no underlying cardiovascular or thrombotic risk factors.[10] In a busy medical practice, is it always possible to consider a patient's personal and family history?

The big 'C'

It's been known since the 1930s, when it was first synthesised, that oestrogen had carcinogenic properties and could cause cancer of the endometrium. An oestrogen-only Pill would increase a woman's risk of endometrial cancer twenty-fold. In an attempt to reduce this risk no currently available form of hormonal contraception uses synthetic oestrogen alone, instead they're either a combination of synthetic oestrogen and progesterone or progesterone alone.

However, in large-scale studies of hormone replacement therapy synthetic progestogens were found to be even more carcinogenic than oestrogen. Progesterone levels are highest during pregnancy and, although it's rare to develop breast cancer at that time, when it does happen, it can spread with the speed of an abscess. New research using breast cancer cells has discovered that progesterone encourages breast cancers to spread rapidly and metastasise.[11]

> *I went into shock when the doctor told me I had breast cancer. I couldn't believe it. I had to have my right breast completely removed and then have radiotherapy, which made me really sick. I continue to ask myself, what could I have done to not get this? I've researched a lot and have become quite an expert. For one thing I wouldn't have taken the Pill for fifteen years.*
>
> **MARILYN, 45**

The synthetic progesterone in Depo-Provera™ causes the most rapid proliferation of breast cancer cells experimentally. Similarly, a study of women who had used progesterone-only pills found a 60 per cent increase in their risk of breast cancer after less than a year of use.

It was in the early 1970s that researchers first began to study the link between oral contraceptive use and breast cancer. Since then a great many studies have found a clear and adverse relationship. A study into cancer and steroid hormones found all of the women diagnosed with breast cancer under 25 years of age and nearly all of those diagnosed under 44 years of age had used combined oral contraceptives.

A large analysis of oral contraceptive studies, published in the medical journal *The Lancet*, found that the use of the Pill before age twenty doubles the risk of breast cancer. Consider the implications of this given that the majority of women who have used the Pill began to take it before they turned twenty.[12]

The greatest risk of breast cancer for women who have ever taken the Pill is if they have a family history of breast or ovarian cancer, if they took the Pill before 1975 or before their first full-term pregnancy. However, even for women who have none of these additional factors, simply using the Pill will increase their risk.

> The best protection against cancer is developing good general health habits and avoiding known carcinogens.

As we have already seen, numerous studies have found an association between the Pill and liver cancer, and the situation is similar with cervical cancer. A study of 47 000 women whose health had been monitored for several decades found that those who had taken the Pill had a *significantly* higher incidence of cervical cancer than those who had never used it, and it's more common the longer a woman took it.[13] Not surprisingly, women who are on the Pill are also more likely to have an abnormal pap smear.

Based on the weight of these and other research findings the World Health Organization's cancer research group, the International Agency for Research on Cancer, announced in July 2005 that it had reclassified the Pill from 'possibly carcinogenic to humans' to 'carcinogenic to humans'. This places the Pill in the same category as tobacco and asbestos—a Class 1 Carcinogen. Perhaps we may soon see packets of the Pill carrying warnings and grim photos similar to those found on cigarettes.

The good news if you take the Pill is that it has a protective effect against the risk of ovarian cancer. Invasive ovarian cancer will generally afflict eight women per hundred thousand woman-years, but among Pill users the rate drops to four women per hundred thousand woman-years.[14]

> We may soon see packets of the Pill carrying warnings and grim photos similar to those found on cigarettes.

In fact, anything that reduces the overall frequency of ovulation—like full-term pregnancy and breastfeeding—

impacts your risk of ovarian cancer. However, in the same way that you're unlikely to plan your babies and breastfeeding around your concern about ovarian cancer, it's unlikely you'd use hormonal contraception for this reason either. The best protection against all kinds of cancer is developing good general health habits and avoiding known carcinogens.

CHAPTER 9

ON THE PILL AND PREGNANT— WHEN THE PILL FAILS

At 25 Jennifer is enjoying her career as a graphic artist and clearly doesn't want to worry about babies yet. She's been living with her boyfriend Mitch for a couple of years and has been on the Pill since she was 21. Jennifer is happy with her contraception because, 'I can be completely relaxed during sex as I'm not at all worried about becoming pregnant.'

Like Jennifer you might be taking the Pill, and putting up with side-effects, because you've been told it provides near-perfect protection against pregnancy. Unfortunately, this is not at all the case. Failure rates quoted in Pill leaflets are around 0.2 to 1 pregnancies per 100 woman-years. This is the 'perfect-use' rate and it relates to when the Pill is used *perfectly* in laboratory conditions. However, 'user' failures—that is, women using the Pill in real, everyday situations—can be as high as 6.2 per 100 woman-years.[1] This means six or more pregnancies per hundred women on the Pill for one year. Based on this statistic, if 100 women use the Pill over a ten-year period we would expect *60 or so* unplanned pregnancies.

If you're on the Pill for its contraceptive effectiveness, consider the results of this research. A recent Australian study of women aged eighteen to 39 on the Pill who weighed 70 kilos or more found that they were 60 per cent more likely to have their birth control Pills fail than women who weighed less. In Australia the *average* woman weighs 66.6 kilograms, so many women just a little heavier than average fall into this category, especially if they've gained weight while on the Pill. A professor of epidemiology, Dr Victoria Holt, says because women who weigh more have a faster metabolic rate they need higher levels of hormones to prevent pregnancy. Another possible cause, she says, is that 'the hormones in birth-control pills are fat soluble and stay in the woman's fat stores so they are not where they need to be—in the bloodstream—in order to work'.[2]

> If you're on the Pill and taking large doses of Vitamin C (over two grams a day), the synthetic hormones will metabolise differently and make your body react as if the hormone dose is higher. When you stop taking the Vitamin C your body will then react as if the Pill has been stopped and its contraceptive effect will no longer be reliable.

Another study found that in a group of 175 'overweight or obese' adolescent girls receiving Depo-Provera™ shots every three months for an eighteen-month period, eighteen, or just over one in ten, became pregnant.[3]

It's estimated that each year almost two million of the more than 60 million women in the United States and Europe who use the Pill become pregnant because of missed Pills—with an average of three missed Pills per month.[4] And, six out of ten women in an Australian study were using contraception when they had an unplanned conception. Of these 43 per cent were on the Pill.[5]

Jessie went on the Pill at thirteen for period pain and heavy bleeding and remained on it until she was 37. During that time she had four unplanned pregnancies. 'I just thought I was very fertile,' she says. Despite this, years of depression and two attempted suicides Jessie was led to believe the Pill was still the best contraception for her. Now, off the Pill and beginning to feel very different in herself, Jessie is enjoying her family—four children and husband Richard—in a way she was never able to before.

> The Pill changes how your body metabolises nutrients so that your nutritional balance is adversely affected while you're on it and for some time afterwards.
> A pregnancy begun under these conditions is far from optimum.

Many modern methods of contraception, especially the Pill and IUD, blur the distinction between abortion and contraception and work by preventing the development of a conception that's taken place—effectively terminating it—as well as by preventing conception itself. Most women seeking abortion today *were using contraception* at the time of conception. In Australia one in three women have had at least one abortion, and in the United Kingdom one in three have had one or more by the time they're thirty. Globally, an estimated 50 million abortions are performed each year.[6]

> Most women seeking abortion today were using contraception at the time of conception.

Often because of the objections of the small pro-life lobby, women keep quiet about abortion and public perception of the effectiveness of contraception becomes distorted. And, let's face it, whatever you think about women's right to choose, abortion can still be confronting. Faced with an unplanned pregnancy you might—perhaps

During the twenty
years Jessie was on
the Pill she had
four unplanned
pregnancies.

with your partner—consider your options: keeping and raising the child, adoption or termination. While many unplanned pregnancies happily go on to be wanted children, this isn't always desirable or possible.

If you find yourself with an unplanned pregnancy and are feeling confused about what you want to do, it may be useful for you to speak with a skilled, objective counsellor who can help you think through your feelings and options.

We highly, *highly* recommend that if you do choose hormonal contraception you do so after carefully considering all your options (and if you know you can use it *perfectly*). Otherwise you may prefer to use something equally, or more, effective and not expose yourself to all the side-effects.

The Pill and your baby

When you take the Pill to avoid pregnancy and pregnancy happens anyway, there are detrimental effects on your and your baby's health. Equally, if you go off the Pill *in order to get pregnant* and this happens quickly, you're still vulnerable to the same adverse effects.

The Pill changes how your body metabolises nutrients and so your nutritional balance is adversely affected while you're on it and for some time afterwards. These deficiencies and imbalances are such that a pregnancy begun under these conditions is far from optimum. Of particular concern are folic acid and zinc as these nutrients are absolutely essential for healthy foetal development.

Levels of folic acid are considerably reduced in Pill users. Maternal deficiency in folic acid has been linked to an *up to five times* greater chance of giving birth to a child with limb defects, and an increased incidence of congenital abnormalities including, neural tube defects resulting in conditions like spina bifida, and Down syndrome. Women who conceive within six months of taking the Pill have been shown to have lower than normal red blood cells and plasma folate levels in the first trimester of pregnancy. Deficiency may also lead to repeated miscarriage.[7]

Zinc is necessary for proper formation of elastin chains in connective tissue. Zinc-deficient women develop stretch marks, have perineums which don't stretch but tear—or need cutting—have nipples which crack readily and have prolonged labours. This is because zinc-deficient women have gaps in their uterine membrane and this compromises its ability to contract. Adequate zinc is essential to maintain the correct ratio of copper to zinc in the body. Many researchers have linked postnatal depression to high copper levels that have failed to return to normal after the birth *because of insufficient zinc.*[8]

Zinc-deficient babies have also been shown to cry excessively and are frequently inconsolable and jittery. This coupled with a depressed zinc-deficient mum is a traumatic, even dangerous, recipe.

I had so wanted this baby but when she cried so much and I was sleeping so little I was anxious all the time and I just wanted it all to go away.
ELLA, 35

Zinc is intimately involved in the correct formation and functioning of a child's immune system, brain, skeletal muscle and bones. In Australia one child in five suffers from asthma, which is an immune dysfunction. This is double the number of children who had asthma thirty years ago. Maternal zinc depletion has also been found to be associated with foetal growth retardation and many types of congenital abnormalities, especially among baby boys. Insufficient zinc can lead to learning and behaviour problems such as attention deficit disorder and attention deficit hyper-activity disorder. Boys are ten times more likely to be affected by these than girls as they need five times more zinc because of their testicular tissue development.

> Zinc-deficient babies cry excessively and are frequently inconsolable and jittery.

It's interesting to note that many of the conditions that result from zinc deficiency in babies and mothers have increased dramatically with the widespread use of the Pill. In addition zinc deficiency compromises folic acid absorption, now recognised as so important for preventing problems with foetal neural tube development.

The Pill also reduces your selenium levels. Selenium has been shown to reduce the chances of foetal deformity, including Down syndrome. This protective effect is lost in pregnancies begun while on the Pill or soon after stopping.

While folate, zinc and selenium are especially important, they're not alone—the whole nutritional spectrum needs to be balanced and at sufficient levels for a healthy pregnancy and baby.

The hormones contained in the Pill may also have a direct and adverse effect on the growing baby and this is particularly problematic if the mother is unaware she is pregnant and continues to take the Pill after conception. It's been estimated that up to three women per hundred who are taking the Pill conceive and, not realising, continue to take it. Research has found the side-effects of taking the Pill during early pregnancy to include foetal limb deformities, heart defects and abnormalities of the reproductive organs. The latter may not become apparent until the child is an adult and has difficulties with his or her own fertility.[9]

There's a much higher incidence of stillbirth, miscarriage and birth defects in pregnancies started while on the Pill or within a month of stopping Pill use, and women who have *at any stage* taken the Pill have an increased chance of giving birth to a child with an obvious defect.[10]

The mini-Pill, which doesn't generally suppress ovulation but causes changes in the endometrium and cervical mucus, also interferes with the passage of eggs or sperm in the Fallopian tubes. This means there's a greater likelihood of a pregnancy being ectopic if conception occurs while on the mini-Pill. If the mini-Pill is taken during breastfeeding, as is common, the breastfeeding baby is likely to suffer all the same nutrient deficiencies as their mum. Synthetic progesterone is also known to act on the hypothalamus, and may masculinise a female infant while she is forming her hormone receptor sites soon after birth increasing her chances of suffering polycystic ovarian syndrome, acne, obesity and infertility; it may also contribute to neonatal jaundice. And researchers recently found that women who took certain types of Pill within a year prior to conceiving increased the risk that their baby boys would have allergic rhinitis, or hay fever.[11]

> Of concern is the huge rise in childhood allergies, diabetes and learning and behaviour problems such as attention deficit disorder and attention deficit hyperactivity disorder.

I put on a lot of weight after I had the contraceptive injection. I'd been slowly losing it before I got pregnant but my doctor wondered if the Depo-Provera™ had contributed to my gestational diabetes.

MEENA, 35

Because there's a link between oral contraceptive use and diabetes, previous Pill use may well be a contributing factor in gestational diabetes, that is, diabetes which occurs during pregnancy. There may also be a link between the Pill's tendency to increase blood pressure and toxaemia in pregnancy.[12]

Epigenetics

New research in the field of genetics has found that we inherit the effects of our parents' and grandparents' lifestyle along with their genes. This is called epigenetics. In particular the effects of hormone-disrupting chemicals such as pesticides have been shown to cross generations.[13] Since the Pill certainly qualifies as hormone-disrupting, we need to be aware that the effects of taking it *at any time* may be passed down to our children, and may be compounding in babies whose mothers and grandmothers have taken it. The extent of these intergenerational effects may just be starting to emerge.

Clearly it's best not to get pregnant on the Pill or soon after. With epigenetics we may soon find that it's best to have never been on it at all. However, for now, if you're at a stage of life when you're not really planning a baby but it's OK if it happens then it's better to use non-chemical contraception.

If you're planning a pregnancy, to avoid the negative repercussions of the Pill for yourself and your baby, we recommend that you use natural contraception for a *minimum* of four months while *actively* undertaking a good pre-conception healthcare program. This includes the prospective father and ensures optimum conditions for conception, pregnancy, trouble-free birth and a beautiful healthy baby.

CHAPTER 10

OFF THE PILL BUT WHERE'S THE BABY? WHEN THE PILL AFFECTS FERTILITY

Often women who go off the Pill ready to have a baby find their cycles and fertility slow to bounce back—sometimes they never do.

Before Suman went on the Pill she had a regular cycle of 28 to 29 days. When she and her husband decided it was time to start their family she stopped taking it. However, getting pregnant proved not to be so easy. Suman says, 'I have been off the Pill for a year now and my cycle is around 35–40 days. My last cycle was 52 days!' Distressed, she adds, 'Which of course is just horrible when you're trying to get pregnant'.

The Pill works by making you temporarily infertile. However, there are many ways in which hormonal contraception can affect your fertility

> They found that nearly a quarter of women trying to conceive couldn't for thirteen months or more after stopping the Pill, whereas only one in ten women who had been using non-hormonal methods of contraception had a similar experience.

even after you stop taking it. The Pill affects your general and reproductive health through alterations in your nutritional status, as we've already mentioned. Nutrient deficiencies and hormonal imbalances also affect cervical mucus and all your reproductive organs, including the ovaries, uterus and endometrium, as well as the pituitary gland—the regulator of your whole fertility cycle.

> *My last cycle was 52 days, which of course is just horrible when you're trying to get pregnant.*
> **SUMAN, 31**

Inflammatory conditions, like endometriosis, are worsened by the Pill, and these can affect your fertility too.[1]

Cervical mucus

One of the ways the Pill works is to change cervical mucus production and this effect often lingers after the Pill is stopped—if this happens the medium through which sperm swim along the female reproductive tract may just not be sufficient.

An expert in this field, Professor Erik Odeblad, has studied the cervix for over 40 years. He found that the mucus-producing cells atrophy as a result of oral contraception.[2] Effectively, long-term use of the Pill ages a woman's cervix and the cervical canal becomes narrower. In this way the cervix of a 33-year-old woman becomes like that of a 45-year-old.[3] A narrower, aged cervix with atrophied mucus-producing cells will make conception more difficult for an otherwise fertile woman.

Candida

Women on the Pill tend to have a weakened immune response. And this allows growth of candida and allergic reactions to develop. These can seriously affect fertility and reproductive health.

Once I was off the Pill I was much better in myself, although the thrush took two years to get rid of.

VIVIEN, 30

Candida can significantly worsen during pregnancy due to hormonal activity, and may cause considerable ill health in the mother and adversely affect the child. Allergic reactions can affect your fertility and reproductive health and may be transmitted to your child.[4]

Chlamydia

A sexually transmitted disease that infects the cervix, in most cases chlamydia will have no obvious symptoms. That is, until you want to get pregnant. The growing incidence of chlamydia infection is one of many factors in the overall numbers of people suffering infertility. While the Pill certainly doesn't cause chlamydia, it has been found to be more common in women who are on the Pill. This is thought to be because of changes to the acidity of the vagina that offers a more receptive environment for infection.[5 & 6]

Tests for chlamydia should be included when fertility problems present themselves as it can be dealt with using appropriate medications. However the longer a woman has been infected, and the more frequently she's been reinfected, the more likely it is that she will have other fertility problems, like blocked Fallopian tubes.[7]

Hormonal balance

Hormonal balance is affected for some time after stopping the Pill. We can see this in the slow return of regular cycles for many women.

> *Prior to being on the Pill for ten years I had very normal cycles and got pregnant easily. After going off it two years ago I haven't had a period. I definitely think the Pill has something to do with it—most of my friends who were on it have some type of fertility problem.*
>
> **ISABELLA, 33**

In a 2004 study, 'time to pregnancy', following long-term combined oral contraception or injectable use was found to be two and three times longer respectively than after condom use—indicating a significant reduction in fertility. The effect was worse the longer the women had used the oral or injectable contraception, or if they were older, obese or already had menstrual disturbances when they started the Pill.[8]

Another study found that nearly a quarter of women trying to conceive couldn't for thirteen months or more after stopping the Pill, whereas only one in ten women using non-hormonal methods of contraception had a similar experience.[9]

Smell and immune system

Fascinating research on women's sense of smell and the Pill gives us an indication of the profound and diverse ways that hormonal contraception can affect us. Women in the most fertile phase of their cycle were found to be the most sensitive to the smell of male sweat, whereas pregnant women had increased sensitivity to food odours during the first few months of pregnancy.

Do you remember our earlier discussion about the hormone mix in the Pill being most similar to the first months of pregnancy? In this study they found that women on the Pill were consistently more sensitive to the smell signalling nourishment—*food!*—and less sensitive to the social smell—*male sweat!*—compared to women not on the Pill.[10] Sounds just like early pregnancy.

> The synthetic hormones alter your hormonal balance to make you temporarily infertile—as if you're already pregnant.

Research has shown that our sense of smell, our own bodily smell and our immune systems are all wired up together and that people are generally attracted to a mate who smells *different* from themselves. When partners who smell different from each other have children, their children have a wider range of immunity than if their parents smelt the same or similar to each other.

Biologist Claus Wedekind researched women on and off the Pill, and who they were sexually attracted to. He found that the Pill reverses the usual smell-immune system signals and that when a woman is on the Pill she tends to choose a mate who has a *similar* immune system. This gives any later children they have together a narrower immunity *and* makes it harder for them to fall pregnant.[11]

> Women in the most fertile phase of their cycle were found to be the most sensitive to the smell of male sweat.

We may wonder if the Pill has influenced a whole generation of women to be with men who have the 'wrong' immune system and who don't smell so good once they're off the Pill. Has this effect on smell contributed to the exponential rise in infertility and divorce figures over the last 40 years?

Connecting fertility problems with the Pill

While many doctors are reluctant to consider that the Pill causes later fertility problems, some women are making this connection themselves. After twelve years on the Pill Sarah doesn't have a period at all without a fertility drug—like Prova™ or Chlomid™—even though she was regular before she took the Pill. Miranda has had really long cycles since going off the Pill, and although her gynaecologist says there's no way that it could still be affecting her, Miranda believes that the Pill's done something to her hormonal balance.

Even when cycles return and are regular after taking the Pill, if they are over 31 days long conception is likely to occur after day seventeen of the cycle. When this happens there is less progesterone support for the pregnancy and miscarriage occurs more frequently. A regular and average length cycle of 27 to 30 days is optimum for a healthy conception.

Those in the fertility drug business seem to be clear about who their customer base is. Fabio Bertarelli, a Swiss billionaire and owner of Serono Laboratories—manufacturer of seven out of ten of the world's fertility drugs—told the *Wall Street Journal*, 'Our usual customers are women over thirty who have been taking birth control pills since they were teenagers or in their early 20s.'[12] Serono Laboratories' success relies on a significant proportion of these women needing fertility drugs to help them conceive. When you think about it, contraception methods based on the idea that your cycles and fertility are a problem, except for the few times when you want to conceive, are by definition not going to be fertility friendly.

Lisa's experience with contraception may sound familiar to you. She says, 'During the years that I struggled with various birth control methods I considered my fertility to be a great big hassle and inconvenience. I never had any interest in pregnancy, childbirth or parenting a kid.' However, she found, 'Once I started charting my cycle I came to make friends with my fertility. I began to really enjoy knowing that I could start a baby during my fertile time if I chose to and became intrigued by the whole idea of being pregnant and giving birth.' Then, she says, 'I conceived when I felt secure enough financially and emotionally to have a child and enjoyed everything about pregnancy, childbirth and nursing my baby.' Like Lisa, using natural methods of contraception can help you to avoid the effects of the Pill on your fertility.

> Contraception methods based on the idea that your cycles and fertility are a problem, except for the few times when you want to conceive, are by definition not going to be fertility friendly.

Francesca Naish is a reproductive expert and naturopath who has all her patients learn fertility awareness methods as part of their pre-conception healthcare program. Not only does this mean they don't need to use hormonal contraception before being ready to conceive, they've also learnt to read their signs of fertility and can time their conception attempts accordingly.

In recognition of the profound effect the Pill, and delayed conception, are having on fertility, government and medical bodies are now recommending that doctors speak with their female patients about 'positive' family planning. That is, considering whether they want children and planning their first conception well before their mid-thirties, if at all possible. Also, that they shouldn't expect that reproductive technologies will automatically deal with any problems that arise. For each couple that receives technological help with their fertility problems and has a healthy baby to take home afterwards, there are many who don't.

CHAPTER 11

MALNUTRITION —A SIDE- EFFECT FOR EVERYONE

As you can see, the side-effects of the Pill are all too numerous and all too commonly experienced by women who take it. In a study of women who had at some time been on the Pill, including current users, three-quarters reported experiencing side-effects and, of these, nearly all had several at once.

> *I felt generally 'low' in the last year of taking the Pill, as if I had lost my sparkle and joy for life. I was also anxious and depressed for the whole ten days before my period.*
> **PENNY, 27**

In addition to side-effects that we have already discussed, the following are commonly experienced by women on the Pill: nausea, vomiting, diarrhoea, urinary tract infection or cystitis, lower genital tract infections, severe weight loss in underweight women, fluid retention and bloating, appetite changes, food cravings and disturbance to blood sugar metabolism possibly contributing to diabetes or hypoglycaemia. Also experienced are eye disorders like double vision, swelling of the optic nerve, contact lens intolerance or grittiness and corneal inflammation, dizziness, fainting and other neurological problems, eczema, skin discolouration, acne, fungal infections and tinea, mouth ulcers, hair loss, facial and body hair growth and varicose veins.

There's a greater tendency for women on the Pill to have allergic reactions like rhinitis, hay fever, asthma and skin rashes, and it can trigger inflammatory conditions of the respiratory, digestive, urogenital, and musculoskeletal systems.[1] In addition, women have expressed feeling 'generally not well', aggressive, angry, vague, irrational, paranoid, 'not clear', 'as if my spirit is blocked' and having 'uncontrollable crying for no apparent reason' while they were on the Pill.[2]

While I was on the Pill I had headaches, thrush and chronic fatigue and I felt moody, vague and depressed. Now, two months after stopping I'm feeling great.

RAE, 25

What causes the side-effects?

There are two major causes of side-effects from the Pill. The first is hormonal—the effects of introduced synthetic hormones washing through your system. The second is nutritional disturbance, caused by the effects of the Pill on your metabolism. As the latter gathers momentum over time many nutrients become depleted and others become overabundant, functionally causing *mal*nutrition. From this many of the other noticeable side-effects kick in or are exacerbated.

The speed and severity of this process for an individual woman will, of course, depend on whether her nutrition was optimal leading up to taking the Pill and her ongoing intake. While optimum nutrition prior to and during Pill use, as well as taking appropriate nutritional supplements,

> The overall nutritional disturbance of the Pill cannot be compensated for.

can certainly help alleviate the overall disturbance, it cannot be fully compensated for as *metabolism itself is affected*.

The insidious symptom creep of Pill-induced malnutrition will vary considerably from woman to woman, as individual tendencies will manifest when general health is compromised. As health problems develop they're often dealt with as unrelated to the Pill, one by one and case by case. However, any treatment that doesn't consider a woman's ongoing use of the Pill will miss a major factor undermining her overall health and exacerbating her particular health issues. Having said that, there are also common side-effects of the Pill that do have particular nutrient profiles, like the relationship between depression and Vitamin B6 and zinc levels.

The Pill affects vitamin, mineral, lipid, essential fatty acid and amino acid metabolism. Vitamins are crucial for all our bodily functions and the vitamins especially affected by the Pill are B6, B12, C, riboflavin, thiamine and folic acid. In the case of B vitamins we find that these plus biotin and B12 can all be compromised if you take the Pill. Reduced Vitamin B1 can lead to you feeling fatigued, weak, experiencing insomnia, vague aches and pains, weight loss, depression, irritability, lack of initiative, constipation, oversensitivity to noise, loss of appetite or sugar cravings, and circulatory problems.[3] When Amanda was on the Pill she found she was tired all the time. Her excitement about her new job quickly disappeared and after a few months she had to cut back her hours to just three days a week. Although she was taking multi-vitamins it wasn't until she was off the Pill for a few months that she really felt like her old self again.

Reduced Vitamin B2 may lead to gum and mouth infections, dizziness, depression, eye irritation, skin problems and dandruff.[4] Julie had always preferred to use contact lenses rather than glasses. She felt freer and less self-conscious. However, when she started taking the Pill she soon found her eyes felt gritty all the time and she had to resort to wearing glasses on a permanent basis.

With Vitamin B6 metabolism disturbed by the Pill you may experience nausea, low stress tolerance, lethargy, anxiety, depression, weakness, nervousness, emotional flare-ups, fatigue, insomnia, mild paranoia, skin eruptions, loss of muscular control, eye problems, herpes and oedema, impaired libido and impaired blood clot prevention.[5] While she was on the Pill Aphrodite felt emotional and anxious all the time. Very soon after she stopped taking it she found her usual clarity and happy disposition returned, much to her great relief.

Since biotin is important in managing candida, when the Pill affects its metabolism and insufficient biotin is available, your body may not be able to control candida levels. A candida overgrowth can lead to a whole raft of unpleasant symptoms, like sugar cravings, overall itchiness, allergies and asthma, chronic fatigue, anxiety and headaches.

When the Pill upsets your Vitamin B12 levels you may experience anaemia, a sore tongue and depression. It's not surprising that depression and mood disorders are among the most commonly experienced side-effects of the Pill as so many of the vitamins that are disturbed are critical for our psychological health.

With reduced Vitamin C levels it may be harder for your body to produce sex hormones when you come off the Pill.[6] This can have multiple effects on your fertility, libido and general sense of well-being. Maggie took the Pill for just a few months but found she felt so 'weird' and unlike her usual happy self that she threw the packet away. 'The last thing I felt like was sex anyway,' she says.

Amanda was tired all the time. Her excitement about her new job quickly disappeared and after a few months she had to cut back her hours to just three days a week.

Minerals are vital to your health as they're critical for many of your essential bodily functions. Some of those that are particularly disturbed by taking the Pill are magnesium, potassium, copper, zinc and selenium. When your magnesium and potassium levels are disrupted you may experience premenstrual symptoms, lumpy breasts, muscle cramps, anxiety, sleeplessness, chocolate or sugar cravings and cardiovascular problems.[7] With insufficient selenium caused by the Pill a pregnancy begun during or soon after taking it diminishes the protective effect selenium offers against deformity and Down syndrome.[8]

> It's not surprising that depression and mood disorders are among the most commonly experienced side-effects of the Pill as so many of the vitamins that are disturbed are critical for our psychological health.

Copper levels are often *increased* on the Pill and can lead to you experiencing immune dysfunction, insomnia, mental turmoil, mood swings, irritability, depression, migraine, hair loss, high blood pressure and clotting tendencies.[9] Jennifer says she became so paranoid on the Pill she was imaging all kinds of crazy things. Now she can see them for what they were but they seemed so *real* to her at the time.

Taking the Pill reduces your absorption of zinc, which can contribute to you developing diabetes, sugar cravings, loss of appetite, poor resistance to infection, skin infections, lowered fertility, impaired normal growth, cell division and tissue repair. Insufficient zinc can also be a big problem for fertility and healthy pregnancy and birth, as you read about in the last chapter.

Irena found out years after the birth of her daughter that low zinc was implicated in many of the features of her experience: a torn perineum, cracked nipples, a fretful, irritable baby and post-natal depression. If she'd known at the time that she could have been zinc deficient after ten years on the Pill she would not have become pregnant so soon after stopping and would have taken steps to restore all her nutritional levels. 'I really could have done without the incredible struggle of that period of my life', she remembers.

A full list of the vitamins and minerals disturbed by taking the Pill and the multiple effects this can have on your health appears in Appendix 2. If you are using any form of hormonal contraception check it out to see if some of what you're experiencing may be related to your contraception. When you consider all the side-effects of the Pill you may find that it starts to look a lot less convenient and easy and much more worrying and tedious.

> *Some of my close friends have decided to trash the Pill and switch to more hormone-friendly methods of birth control. All of them have reported that they are much more mentally sound, are having fewer fights with their boyfriends and that they feel more energetic.*
> **BELINDA, 22**

Very often a woman experiencing unacceptable side-effects of the Pill will be offered another brand, or another type of hormonal contraception.

While there are some differences in the formulation and delivery of various types of hormonal contraception, and it might be that one type suits a particular woman *somewhat* more than another, these differences are relatively minor—although they may be exaggerated for marketing purposes. Often a woman just exchanges one set of side-effects for another. When Katrina switched to Diane 35™ she felt more emotional around her withdrawal bleed and had an unwanted increase in breast size. She did like, however, the improvement in her skin. For Kate it wasn't until after she moved and changed doctor that her new doctor said the Pill may be the cause of her nausea, fatigue and headaches and changed her formulation. Her symptoms improved, although she still had them some of the time.

Emma had been on and off the Pill since she was sixteen years old, primarily to help her manage painful periods and heavy bleeding. Over the past fourteen years she had tried most brands at some time or another, including the mini-pill and Depo-Provera™. Her side-effects included depression, headaches, cramping, mood swings as well as violent and continuous nausea leading to massive weight loss. However, things did improve with Implanon™, 'although it does dull my libido', she admits, 'but perhaps that's a good thing at the moment with no relationship on the horizon'. For Emma Implanon™ *has* made a difference and she is happier with this therapy than those she'd tried before. Nonetheless we need to remember that nutritional disruption will gradually erode general health over time *for everyone*. When she's ready Emma would be better off seeking therapies that can heal and balance her underlying hormonal condition and support her general health and wellbeing.

> *The three-month shots really affected my state of mind and I became unhappy and destructive in my relationship, ultimately resulting in a break-up.*
>
> EMMA, 30

Sometimes a doctor will use the placebo effect by offering you the same formulation in the guise of a different brand name in the hope of alleviating side-effects. The placebo effect is understood to occur when a doctor gives us 'medicine' for a particular condition and that condition improves although the medicine contained no active ingredients. In these situations it's actually our *faith* in the doctor and medicine that heals us. Many doctors find this effective and it's been estimated that four out of ten doctors use the placebo effect in their medical practice.[10] So, in relation to the Pill, the placebo effect may be attempted by switching one brand of Pill for another, even though their active ingredients are the same.

> *I still have most of the symptoms some of the time.*
>
> KATE, 25

Whether a new brand of Pill or a different delivery of hormones is the same formulation or a different one it still needs to be strong enough to override your natural fertility cycle and induce temporary infertility. All hormonal contraception is either a combination of synthetic oestrogen and progesterone, or synthetic progesterone alone, delivered orally via pills, under the skin via injection or implant, through the skin via a patch, vaginally via a vaginal ring or in-utero via hormone impregnated IUDs. There are only a few possible configurations of these variables and swapping them about is much like rearranging deckchairs on the *Titanic*, as the saying goes. Whatever the configuration, your health and wellbeing are at risk and may start to sink and, as with the *Titanic*, you won't necessarily see it coming.

> Through its profound hormonal impact the Pill may also be interfering with the fundamental chemistry of who we are and what we can become.

CHAPTER 12

ARE PERIODS REALLY BAD FOR YOU?

According to some experts periods are bad for your health and the most natural approach is to suppress them altogether with continuous use of the Pill. We have a long history of negative attitudes towards menstruation and the assumption is often made that women would do without it if they could. Seeing a marketing opportunity, the pharmaceutical industry is now selling us menstrual suppression.

'To have so many periods', Dr Elismir Coutinho, author of *Is Menstruation Obsolete?* argues, 'isn't only a nuisance, but may be an unnecessary hazard to a woman's emotional and physical health'. As it happens, Coutinho was also part of the team who developed Depo-Provera™, the injectable contraceptive that suppresses a woman's period for three months at a time.[1]

Following the same theme in 2003 Barr Laboratories released Seasonale™ in the United States. A contraceptive pill packed as 84 hormone pills followed by seven placebo pills, Seasonale™ allows a woman four withdrawal bleeds a year instead of the usual twelve or thirteen. This was the first extended-cycle contraceptive pill on the market. It was promoted with the slogan 'fewer periods, more possibilities' and, curiously, as the pill to reduce the number of periods a year to a more 'natural' number. In the twelve months up to June 2006 sales for Seasonale™ reached a cool US$120 million. Now, a new menstrual suppression regime has been released by Wyeth Pharmaceuticals as Anya™ in the United States and Canada, and Lybrel™ in Britain. These hormone pills are designed to be taken 365 days a year to 'put women in control of when *or if* they want to menstruate'.

It's been four years now since I came off the Pill and menstruation has become a special time for me—like a mystical feminine ritual.
CHARLEY, 27

In this way menstrual suppression is being recommended for menstrual problems and as a lifestyle choice for women who don't like periods or find them inconvenient. As is often the case the reality of taking hormones for menstrual suppression is not the same as the image presented by product advertising. Studies of women on both Depo-Provera™ and Lybrel™ found that unscheduled, breakthrough bleeding and spotting lasting four or five days was a very common experience. In this way a predictable bleed is foregone and is replaced by an unpredictable one. Even for a woman not wanting a period is this really an improvement?

Menstrual suppression is also sold as a therapy to eliminate the mood swings and discomfort associated with periods, but as we already know, these drugs come with their own raft of side-effects and, as you will soon see, there are many therapeutic and lifestyle approaches to hormonal problems that lead to a healthy menstrual experience without all the side-effects. Sophie was put on the Pill to treat her heavy, painful periods when she was fifteen. While her symptoms eased somewhat other effects from the Pill troubled her. Basically, she just didn't feel like her normal self. Trying another approach which involved adjusting her diet, a few sessions of acupuncture and learning some helpful yoga poses soon made all the difference to her menstrual experience. Sophie now enjoys 'a special relationship with the natural cycles and seasons'.

For all the hoo-hah around the release of drugs for menstrual suppression, it's simply a repackaging of the Pill to extend its market. The Pill has always suppressed the menstrual cycle and periods on the Pill have only ever been withdrawal bleeds. What has changed is the packaging of the active hormone pills relative to the placebo pills.

I like having a period because it's an excuse not to be so busy trying to do everything at once—I love to go slow for a couple of days.

FRAN, 20

About menstrual suppression the experts—doctors, feminists, bioethicists and women themselves—are bitterly divided. On the one hand, advocates say, it's all about providing women with choices and giving them control. We've already been manipulating Mother Nature for decades, so why stop now? But detractors say menstrual suppression is a reckless and profit-driven enterprise, or, as one women's health expert calls it, 'the largest uncontrolled experiment in the history of medical science, hands down'.[2]

Dr Leslie Miller, a professor of obstetrics and gynaecology at the University of Washington, runs a pro-suppression website—www. Noperiod.com—and her view is that, 'there's nothing natural about menstruation' and that with menstrual suppression, 'every day your hormones are the same. It's a modern problem to have thirteen periods a year for 35 years.' Dr Miller goes on to say she thinks the continuous Pill is a 'modern solution to a modern problem'. If you find her definition of 'natural' curious, you may like to take a look at how she elaborates her argument on her website.

On the other hand endocrinologist Dr Jerilynn Prior believes that menstruation is an amazingly intricate, carefully crafted cycle and is a vital sign of our health. 'To wantonly disrupt it is a horrifying thought', she says, 'the continuous-use Pill is just a way for pharmaceutical companies to revive flagging products—to find fresh ways to market them by giving them a new face and a new name'.[3]

When I was travelling I tried to honour my blood by staying in one place and treating myself to slightly more opulent accommodation. One time I was in Thailand and found a beautiful bungalow set in exquisite gardens for a great off-peak price. I spent three days there feeling like a queen in my little palace, like I was celebrating my womanhood.

TARA, 32

Geraldine Matus, a holistic reproductive healthcare practitioner from Edmonton in Canada, adds, 'From a cultural perspective, I think it's misogynistic. Women's bodies are a marvellous thing to commodify. We have all sorts of processes that can be turned into diseases and disease models: pregnancy, nursing, menstruation and menopause. I could make the same argument about men and ejaculation. I could say, "Men don't need to ejaculate. It's messy; it means a loss of essential nutrients; it's embarrassing when you have a wet dream. So take a pill to suppress it." But that would change everything about how a man works . . . that's how ridiculous *this* is.'

Women's conflicted feelings about menstruation—the mess, the fuss, the pain—are stoked by centuries, if not millennia, of superstition that has, in many ways, reinforced the perception of women as the 'weaker' sex. This has often caused women to despise their own cycles. Feminist writers have also largely ignored this issue, not wanting to draw attention to what they've also perceived to be a feminine weakness.

When Rebecca came off the Pill at 26 after ten years of taking it, she felt as if she was beginning to listen to her body, as a woman, for the first time. She says, 'It was as if I became a woman when I started to experience, and I must say enjoy, my own natural cycle for the first time in so many years'. She adds, 'I also felt angry that the Pill was given to me so young with *no-one* advising me about its far-reaching effects and what I would be losing'.

The pharmaceutical company Wyeth's own research found that nearly two-thirds of women expressed interest in giving up their periods. This is mirrored in similar research undertaken by Linda Andrist, who coordinates the women's health program at the Institute of Health Professions in Boston. She found that women don't want to confront their bodily functions anymore, that 'we're too busy'.[4] Other research has found that many women view their periods as a symbol of fertility and health and that women have a complex love-hate relationship with their cycles.[5]

> As I became in touch with my cycle I realised I didn't want to do much when
> I'm bleeding. I've organised my life around these needs and I now experience
> a joy-filled, complication free, intuitive bleeding time.
>
> CAROLINE, 28

However, several studies have turned up other, rather enlightening findings on this subject. When symptoms generally attributed to women and the menstrual cycle—mood swings, depression, energy fluctuations, food cravings, headaches, mental confusion and bloating—were recorded over monthly time-periods *by men and women*, and eliminating sex-specific symptoms like breast tenderness, it was found that the men in the study reported these symptoms *at least as often* as the women. Strong variations occurred between individuals but not between the sexes overall.[6] These results suggest that troubling menstrual symptoms are more a result of overall depleted health than of the menstrual cycle per se.

Despite this, menstrual suppression is most often touted as a way to eliminate menstrual problems. However, synthetic hormones can *never* balance your hormones; at best they can mask your symptoms by effectively smashing the warning light your menstrual problems represent. While these can certainly be debilitating, they are nonetheless eminently treatable with nutrition, lifestyle and hormone balancing therapies. Once treated a *healthy* menstrual cycle can emerge that, for many women, is a profoundly satisfying experience of their femininity and sexuality.

Nicola found that once she came off the Pill she felt 'much more alive, much more in tune with my body and my senses'. She feels that her intuition is returning, as far as knowing what may be causing physical symptoms, and that she's in a much better position to make decisions about her health that are right for her. Now, having received naturopathic treatment for the debilitating premenstrual symptoms she had suffered for years, she really appreciates the gentle rhythm of her changing cycle.

Understanding cyclic changes and working with them in a positive way is not only healthier for women but can also enrich our relationships—the more we understand about how our fertility works the more amazing the whole process and design can appear, and the more the Pill and menstrual suppression becomes counterintuitive.

For adolescent girls experiencing the profound physical and psychological transformation of puberty, the possibility of menstrual suppression carries a very troubling message. How can a girl develop a healthy body image and self-esteem when the natural unfolding processes of her fertility are so centrally devalued and denigrated?

I was at my best friend Molly's house when I got my first period so we celebrated together. I was very proud—getting my period made me feel very feminine. I think it's amazing how our bodies work.

ROSELLA, 14

CHAPTER 13

WHAT ABOUT YOUR TEENAGE DAUGHTER?

The Pill has become the great cure-all for menstrual and hormonal problems, and is prescribed liberally to soothe our collective fears about teen sexuality and pregnancy. Of the 90 per cent of Western women who have at some time taken the Pill, a great many started before their eighteenth birthday. Some were as young as twelve.[1 & 2]

Maybe you were put on the Pill as a teenager yourself? And you may well have experienced some relief from your troubling symptoms. Sue's dad was a doctor and when she started to have extreme period pain he gave her Valium and then put her on the Pill. This helped, although Sue's memories of her middle teen years are of spending quite a bit of time lying around in a drug haze. Some years later when she decided she didn't want her cycle regulated by the Pill, or to take painkillers anymore, Sue found other ways to ease her pain and now enjoys her periods symptom free.

The younger a girl is when she goes on the Pill the more likely it's been prescribed for therapeutic purposes—for irregular periods, heavy periods, period pain, polycystic ovarian syndrome, acne—or even simply to eliminate periods. Using the Pill to regulate periods is, however, a misunderstanding of the action of the Pill and of the intricacies of the menstrual cycle. Many girls' cycles can naturally take two years or so to settle into a regular pattern after their onset. If irregularity persists or is distressing there are many effective alternative therapies that can help to establish hormonal balance. The Pill, on the other hand, *eliminates* the natural menstrual cycle and replaces it with a false state like early pregnancy, interrupted at regular intervals by a withdrawal bleed during the placebo pill days. Even the mini-Pill—which doesn't prevent ovulation—regulates the menstrual cycle with synthetic hormones and inhibits a girl's body from achieving its own natural hormonal balance.

> The Pill artificially regulates the cycle, supporting an unnatural situation and masking what's underlying it. If there's a blood deficiency the Pill will make a withdrawal bleed happen—contrary to what a woman's body would naturally be able to do.
>
> DANIEL SAULWICK, TRADITIONAL CHINESE MEDICINE PRACTITIONER

While heavy periods, period pain, polycystic ovarian syndrome and acne can certainly be distressing and many girls have gratefully taken the Pill hoping to alleviate these symptoms when nothing else is offered, nonetheless the Pill cannot solve the underlying problem.

At her mum's suggestion Ruby was put on the Pill when she was fourteen for heavy periods and cramps. At fifteen she was struggling with depression and was sent to a psychiatrist who recommended antidepressants. Much as she wanted relief Ruby was reluctant to take more drugs and a family friend suggested a different approach. She began having weekly acupuncture and counselling sessions as well as taking therapeutic herbs. After a few months, Ruby went off the Pill and while her cycles took four months to become regular again, her menstrual symptoms were greatly reduced. And, most importantly, Ruby felt stronger and happier in herself.

Contraception

The other reason teenagers go on the Pill is, of course, for contraception. Either a girl who is considering, or is in, a sexual relationship will visit a doctor for the Pill to manage this step in her life responsibly, or her parents, guardian or doctor may put her on the Pill 'just in case'. Certainly availability of contraception is critical for those wanting to explore sexual relationships, and unplanned teen pregnancy is best avoided wherever possible. However, the effort to manage this complex situation has at times resulted in oversimplified, heavy-handed and dangerous solutions. In this way we expose girls to myriad physical and emotional problems at a time in their life when they may not yet know themselves well enough to assess or understand the underlying causes. And as they mature, they only know themselves on the Pill.

Young women who have been on the Pill and decide to seek other contraceptive methods rarely, if ever, report having received sufficient information about the Pill, adequate check-ups or information about alternatives. In other words, they're not able to make truly informed choices. Sexually active teenagers do undoubtedly need effective contraception, however, the assumption that this should be the Pill, in the form of a tablet or an injection or implant that can be forgotten, belies the *range* of effective contraception available, including those that have no side-effects.

> The Pill eliminates the natural menstrual cycle and replaces it with a false state of early pregnancy.

At sixteen I was in my first sexual relationship and went on the Pill. I thought it was the only form of contraception available. My boyfriend and I both felt that we were being responsible. After I started taking it I had a lot of emotional confusion and this eventually led to my relationship breaking down. Now, after coming off the Pill I feel a lot more energetic and optimistic in my life. My anxiety levels have gone right down and I'm happier.

ROSIE, 21

Best practice

The accepted best practice in paediatric medicine is to start from the least invasive therapy and to move cautiously to those that are more invasive, and only as absolutely necessary. This common sense approach acknowledges that drugs and medical procedures, while they can of course be very helpful, do have undesirable or dangerous side-effects and all the more so for young bodies.

In direct contrast to this young girls are often given the Pill on the first presentation of menstrual or hormonal problems—like acne, irregular, heavy or painful periods or polycystic ovarian syndrome—despite there being a variety of effective non-invasive treatments for these. In a study of women who had at some time been on the Pill or used other hormonal contraception, one-third began before their seventeenth birthday, close to half before their eighteenth and fully eight out of ten before they left their teens.[3] Clearly the Pill is a drug of first choice when treating girls rather than one cautiously and carefully considered.

I went on the Pill at sixteen and although I had terrible mood swings—I cried a lot and was often angry and very emotional, and had enlarged veins on my legs— I didn't realise till later any of this was to do with the Pill and just got my repeat scripts over the phone.

RENA, 23

A heavy chemical load for young bodies

From this last statistic we can see that a great many of the estimated 300 million women worldwide who have been or still are on the Pill began while not only legally children but, more importantly, when their bodies, and reproductive systems, were still developing. As such they're not only vulnerable to all the usual side-effects—a heavy enough load for any girl or woman—but in addition there are further dangers associated with ongoing use of these drugs from such a young age.

Let's be clear, the Pill carries serious risks to a teenager's health. It's metabolised in the liver and causes more than 150 chemical changes in a girl's body, many of which are still not fully understood.[4]

> *I could never put my finger on what was wrong with the Pill. The woman at Family Planning told me I would be surprised how many girls felt that way.*
> **JENNY, 20**

If a girl who is not ovulating regularly goes on the Pill, both menstruation and ovulation may be suppressed permanently, or take much longer, or need treatment, to return. A recent study showed that a third of healthy girls aged eighteen still had anovular menstrual cycles—that is, no ovulation—while nonetheless menstruating regularly.

> *Our usual customers are women over thirty who have been taking birth control pills since they were teenagers or in their early twenties.*
> **FABIO BERTARELLI, MANUFACTURER OF FERTILITY DRUGS**

Heightened risk of fracture

If a girl begins to use the Pill while she's still growing, it may prevent her from reaching her full height as the increased oestrogenic load speeds up the closure of her long bones. A recent US study found that when girls 'at risk of becoming too tall' were given the Pill their growth was effectively stopped but their fertility was also considerably compromised.

The use of Depo-Provera™ injections has been associated with *significant loss of bone mineral density*, increasing with duration of exposure and without necessarily being reversible. During adolescence the usual large gains in bone mass have been found to be slowed down by these hormonal injections as well as some forms of oral contraception. The degree of bone loss—or lack of bone gain—is *more pronounced in adolescence* than in young adult women who typically have smaller changes in bone mass. While relative bone density can be tested for, the outcome of increased brittleness and the heightened risk of fracture doesn't usually manifest until several decades later, by which time the damage has well and truly been done. Like many health problems of advancing age, this is one we are certainly better to prevent than exacerbate.[5]

Heightened risk of cancer

Studies have found that the increased risk of breast cancer among Pill users is predominant in women who used it for at least four years before their first pregnancy. Since the breast tissue of teenage girls is still developing, it's particularly sensitive to overstimulation by synthetic oestrogen. Studies have found that using the Pill before 20 years of age doubles the risk of breast cancer.[6] And one study found that the younger the women were at the time of diagnosis of breast cancer, the greater the possibility that they would be dead within five years.[7]

Another study found that women who started using the Pill at an earlier age were at increased risk of cervical cancer than those who started later. The risk of developing a severe cancer was 50 per cent greater for Pill users as well as for women who had a cervical smear indicating pre-cancerous cells and continued to use the Pill.[8]

Parental consent

The Pill is generally available to teenage girls without parental consent, or without them needing to be informed. The age when this right to privacy kicks in varies from country to country and is often at the discretion of the doctor. While many of us have enjoyed our own right to privacy as teenagers and there are some good reasons to make it available, there is a down side. Teenagers may easily make omissions in giving personal and family history during a medical appointment and this can have serious consequences.

In 1994 when Caroline was fourteen she had a boyfriend and wanted to go on the Pill. She went to her local Family Planning clinic and after a brief consultation she was given a prescription. Soon after she started taking the Pill Caroline began to get headaches, developed numbness to her right side and hands and was seeing flashing lights. She lapsed into a coma for some days and when she regained consciousness she could only move her eyes. She died eleven months later.

Caroline had known circulatory problems but she wasn't asked for her medical history nor warned of the risks associated with taking the Pill, nor did her parents know she had been prescribed the Pill. The Pill aggravated her problems and as a result she lost her life.[9]

Education

Critics of sex education claim that talking with teenagers about sex will lead to increased sexual activity and unplanned pregnancies, however there is no evidence for this. On the contrary, in Western countries where sex education is comprehensive, teen pregnancy is well below that of other Western countries where sex education is restricted, nonexistent or only teaches abstinence. In fact studies have shown that first full sexual experiences occur later where sex education is most comprehensive, as is the case in the Netherlands and Sweden. As an analogy we could say that teaching good nutrition doesn't lead to overeating but rather to greater awareness and better food choices.

I don't think I would have had so many sexual partners if I'd had more knowledge about my body.
RHIANNON, 24

On a global level and across cultures it's been found that the single most powerful way to reduce population growth is to educate women. Availability of contraception alone won't do it and nor will forced sterilisation. However, educating women who are then empowered to plan their lives and families has been shown to make the greatest difference of all. The Chinese one-child policy is perhaps the exception to this, but no other country has as yet been inclined to follow their heavy-handed lead.

Many women who later go off the Pill and as a consequence find a number of their physical and emotional symptoms fading away dearly wish they'd had more information and wider choices from the beginning and not been left to stumble upon them along the way. After thirteen years on the Pill Louise was 29 when she and her husband decided to try fertility awareness methods. She enjoyed learning about her cyclic patterns and found, 'I began to feel really feminine when I tuned into my cycle'. Louise really wishes she'd had this information years before: 'I could have saved myself a lot of emotional pain,' she says regretfully.

Rather than relying on the ease of writing scripts for the Pill to manage teenage contraception we could be investing in ongoing availability of broad-based, non-commercial education with information about contraception, sexual health and fertility. Girls, and boys, could only benefit from a clear intention to create a contraceptively literate generation able to make confident and appropriate decisions for every occasion. The Pill may still be one of the methods on offer but with a full understanding of side-effects and alternatives and as part of an ongoing process of informed choice.

So, what do you do about your teenage daughter?

At the risk of oversimplifying and overgeneralising the issues, it will nonetheless help if you can actively make a positive connection with your daughter as she changes from a little girl into a pubescent one. Through exploring and understanding your own experience of your first period you can offer her a graceful and positive passage into her cyclical life. You can support her ongoing learning about her cycle and healthy ways to manage it. As her interest in boys deepens, keep the communication channels open in a non-judgemental, non-fearful way.

> *I talk to my mum about everything. It's good to have someone to talk to who knows stuff and who's been through it all 'cause your friends don't know any better than you.*
>
> **CHARLEY, 19**

Throughout this process—no less a journey for a parent—seek to be well informed, including consulting helpful health professionals. When it comes to contraception, at whatever age this need arises, if you've kept communication between you open and supportive, you'll have an active role in helping your daughter work out what's best for her. At the very least you'll have provided her with a positive model of how to go about making her own informed choice.

> *Having suffered depression and a lot of confusion during my teenage years I was determined to offer something different to my daughter. So far, so good. We talk a lot and look at options and strategies together. I feel like we're on a wonderful feminine journey of discovery. For me it's incredibly healing and for her, I don't know . . . for her it's just how it is.*
>
> **IRENA, MOTHER OF THEA, 16**

CHAPTER 14

TAKING THE PILL FOR SKIN AND PERIOD PROBLEMS

Debbie went on the Pill for period pain and heavy bleeding at eighteen. This brought her great relief and allowed her control over her life: she could plan holidays, not need to take time off work and she had contraception. Although she put on a lot of weight and her moods could be foul, she was nonetheless grateful for the relief the Pill gave her. In her late twenties she began to do some personal development work. As she started to address her negative feelings about being a woman and put in place some healthy lifestyle practices, she was able to heal her symptoms and now she really enjoys her natural cycle and has no intention of going back on the Pill.

At 25 Erika was on the Pill for acne. She didn't need contraception at this point, just help for her skin, and the Pill made a big difference.

Like Debbie and Erika you might be using the Pill or considering it for a period problem or a skin condition and don't know any other way to deal with the issue effectively. The Pill is often a doctor's first medicine of choice for treating many period problems such as premenstrual syndrome (PMS), period pain, endometriosis, polycystic ovarian syndrome, irregularity, no period, heavy periods, and fibroids, as well as skin problems. Even girls as young as twelve or thirteen are prescribed it for their menstrual difficulties. The assumption is that synthetic hormones will help to balance your natural ones and create wellbeing, but this is a misunderstanding—in fact they can never balance your hormones.

What is the real cause of menstrual problems?

Maintaining hormonal regulation is something like putting on a complicated stage play with each of the different hormones having different roles to play. Hormones—the microscopic substances carried in the blood and detected by blood tests—are the actors, directors and managers in the monthly play called the menstrual cycle.[1]

RUTH TRICKEY, HERBALIST

Menstruation is a normal, healthy process in women—when it's working well it's an indication of your overall healthiness. When there are difficulties it's like your system is saying to you 'time to put in some extra self-care strategies, you're getting a bit rundown'. Some women have problems such as period pain from the beginning of their menstruating life, suggesting an even greater need for care with their health.

When your menstrual health does take a dive, you need to check out the usual suspects implicated in any health issue, such as poor diet, lack of exercise, the stress of trying to do too much, the stress of living and working in polluted environments (including electromagnetic pollution), as well as the chronic low-grade stress that results from the negativity surrounding periods in general. Some women also have a genetic inheritance, thyroid problems or a poorly functioning immune system, digestion, liver or kidneys, which can all contribute to menstrual distress.

In modern medical practice the cycle itself is often seen as the culprit and it's assumed that if the cycle is switched off, or artificially regulated, then the problem will be solved. For some women and girls the Pill may seem to do just that—make the problem disappear—but this is more akin to smashing the warning light than finding and fixing the underlying cause. Sooner or later the problem will resurface and you may be worse off. Erika's skin condition apparently cleared up on the Pill but what she didn't appreciate was how it was compromising her overall health, and would make her skin pasty and dull over time, even developing brown patches.

> *By removing . . . symptoms with the Pill, this perfect expression of the disordered vitality of the patient is suppressed. And, as a consequence the best possible response of the body is to drive deeper into the interior and throw up much more serious symptoms in order to be heard.*
> **ALASTAIR GRAY, HOMOEOPATH**

If you're using the Pill to handle your PMS, period pain, polycystic ovarian syndrome or acne, it's important to realise that the cause of your symptoms hasn't actually gone away, it's been repressed. However, an absence of symptoms can bring you very necessary relief and give you the space to think about other options, rather like the way antidepressants can get you out of a black hole sufficiently to allow you to initiate changes that will make you feel good without drugs.

Creating further problems

While taking the Pill may seem to ease your menstrual symptoms, when you repress the cycle you can create further difficulties for yourself. These can be poor overall health, feeling unconnected to yourself or what lights you up, moodiness, reactivity and depression, and you might also have more difficulties with your period and fertility when you do come off the drug. As homoeopath Alastair Gray puts it, 'Symptoms are not just the disease but are seen as the manifestation of that disease, the result of the disease. The snow is not the winter. The snow is the result of the winter. By removing these symptoms with the Pill, this perfect expression of the disordered vitality of the patient is suppressed. And, as a consequence, the best possible response of the body is to drive deeper into the interior and throw up much more serious symptoms in order to be heard.'

In the language of Traditional Chinese Medicine, practitioner Jane Lyttleton tells us that the Pill causes symptoms of liver qi (energy) stagnation in some women. This can lead to premenstrual symptoms, headaches and mood changes, and eventually also increase the risk of more substantial symptoms of stagnation like fibroids.

Herbalist Wendy Dumaresq has discovered that if a woman is on the Pill and seeking treatment for any condition 'she can be difficult to treat . . . I can still make a difference but not as much as is otherwise possible'. Dr Claudia Welch has noticed that 'it's more of a challenge to the practitioner to really be able to detect and treat any underlying imbalance in women on the Pill'. In other words, the Pill makes it harder to heal health problems in general and it could be exacerbating your menstrual woes rather than aiding them.

The Pill creates nutritional deficiencies and we all know that good nutrition is one of the fundamental building blocks for good health. It's a contradiction to imagine that the Pill can create long-term wellbeing when it's draining your body of essential nutrients. Making sure you have a good diet while on the Pill is essential even though the Pill will still disturb absorption of key nutrients.

The best way to heal your hormonal problems is to put in place healthy self-care practices slowly and gently, and to be more accepting of your body's cyclical rhythms. Over time this will ease your menstrual problems and you'll feel much better in yourself. You'll also have more energy for the things you love, feel calmer, more focused and positive about life and have glowing skin! *No* drug can give you that kind of high. Later on we'll be looking at things *you* can do to heal your symptoms.

CHAPTER 15

ARE YOU THINKING ABOUT COMING OFF THE PILL?

So, you're thinking of coming off the Pill? Perhaps you're tired of the side-effects and the risks to your health and want to enjoy your natural cycle. Or, maybe you want to experience a more rewarding sex life or are ready to have a baby. There are, of course, important things to consider when you come off the Pill. Women ask, 'Is it OK to stop at any time, or do I have to complete the packet that I'm on? What will I do about contraception when I'm off the Pill? Can I do anything more to support my health to recover from the drug?' And, 'Will my menstrual problems come flooding back?'

Coming off the Pill has made such a difference to how my partner perceives my sexuality and the commitment we both make to contraception.

MELINDA, 33

Stopping the Pill

You can stop taking the combination Pill at any time in the 'cycle' because there's no real cycle to interrupt, similarly, with the Patch™ and vaginal ring. A breakthrough bleed will occur a day or so after. Although this isn't actual menstruation, you can think of it as the first day of your cycle for the purpose of beginning to observe your cycles.

If you're using the mini-Pill you'll need to complete the pack you're on because it doesn't prevent ovulation. So, rather than interrupting the cycle it's best to use your mini-Pill cycle as a blueprint for the natural cycle you want to re-establish. If you are using a LNG-IUD or IUS, have it removed by a trained medical doctor just before your period is due.

If you've been using Depo-Provera™, you'll simply have to wait out its effect and of course not have another! Implants can be removed at any time but it does need to be done by a doctor.

Depending on how long you've been on the Pill and how regular your cycle was before, you may experience some irregularity. For some women it may take months before a regular cycle is re-established, as was the case for the women whose stories are in Chapter 10: 'Off the Pill, but where's the baby? When the Pill affects fertility'. When Louise came off the Pill at nineteen after a year of taking it, her period took a year to return, and when it did, it was irregular. Jessie's period came back heavy and fast— her first one lasted ten days and the next period came three weeks later. Clarissa, who was on the Pill for a year and then tried an implant for three months, established a regular cycle straight away after each. And Abby is still waiting for her period to return twelve months after her last Depo Provera™ injection.

Supporting your health

To help your body recover from the Pill, it's important to have a good healthy lifestyle as we'll describe in Chapter 27: 'The natural way to menstrual wellbeing'. Elimination of the Pill can be sped up with the use of natural remedies to detoxify the system and stimulate the normal functioning of the endocrine glands.[1] Naturopathy, homoeopathy, Traditional Chinese Medicine and Ayurvedic Medicine can all be of great help.

Self-care practices that you can try include drinking dandelion root 'coffee' (without sugar) to encourage elimination from your liver, and nettle tea to nourish your endocrine system.

As the Pill interferes with the absorption of key nutrients, apart from making sure you have an excellent diet, it might be helpful to get yourself a good multi-vitamin and mineral supplement as well as some of those good oils—essential fatty acids. It's also important to have a balance of protein to carbohydrates to support your endocrine health. In other words *don't* overdo the carbs. Have a serving of protein—about the size of the palm of your hand—at every meal. And, of course, avoid white flour and sugar.

When a woman stops the Pill we use acupuncture to re-establish the functioning of certain channels, which have been switched off during the time of Pill use. Treatment usually involves nutritional supplementation to restore normal balance, and herbal, or other naturopathic treatments, for uterine health, normal function of the pituitary/ovarian axis, healthy cervical/mucous membrane/endometrial status, liver support to rid the body of excess hormones and anti-inflammatory remedies.

JANE LYTTLETON, TRADITIONAL CHINESE MEDICINE PRACTITIONER

You might notice your emotions going through some shifts too. You may experience more depth of feeling, which might be really positive or a little overwhelming. Coming off Depo-Provera™ caused a sensory overload for Abby. She became very sensitive to touch, much more emotional and, thankfully, felt her sexual energy come back to life. 'It became incredibly apparent how numb my body had become on the shot. So, I definitely experienced, and am still going through, some psychological side-effects,' she admits. As the effects of the Pill wear off and nutrient metabolism returns to normal, you should, however, notice your emotions settle down, and generally have a greater sense of wellbeing and ease.

If you had PMS or other menstrual problems before you went on the Pill, start practising the self-care strategies that you'll find in Chapters 27 and 28 as soon as possible. Once you're off the Pill you'll be able to explore your own period power, which in itself will start to improve your PMS symptoms.

Taking care of contraception

If you're in a relationship, you may have already discussed stopping the Pill with your partner because, naturally, it's going to have consequences for him too. However, if you haven't yet, and even if it's non-negotiable for you, it's important to share your thoughts about why you're doing it. And you'll need to discuss your ongoing contraception needs, of course. If you're the male partner, you may have been the one to suggest your partner stop taking the Pill because you've seen what it's been doing to her health and moods, or it just hasn't felt right.

Take the time to learn about other methods of contraception, and how to be effectively covered. The contraception you choose and how you use it is all part of your sexuality and relationship. Instead of feeling hassled by contraception we suggest you adopt an attitude of curiosity—enjoy the power you have to make positive and conscious choices.

Wanting to conceive?

You may be coming off the Pill because you want to have a baby; however, it's important that you *don't* try to conceive straight away. Because the Pill has compromised your health, the health of your baby may also be compromised if you conceive before clearing the effects of the Pill from your body. For the optimum health of mother and baby we recommend actively practising pre-conception health care for at least four months prior to conception attempts.

According to Francesca Naish and Jan Roberts, the authors of *The Natural Way to Better Babies*, pre-conception health care involves 'making sure there is an adequate supply of all those factors which are essential to the health of your sperm and ova and to foetal development, and an absence of all those things which have been shown to be harmful'.[2] This includes a healthy diet, supplements, giving up smoking, alcohol, caffeine and drugs, cleaning up your environment, addressing allergies, reducing stress and getting fit. We suggest you read their book for the complete lowdown on pre-conception health care.

You may have had your fertility compromised by the Pill and find it difficult to conceive. As well as practising pre-conception health care and using the resources mentioned above, we strongly recommend you see a specialist naturopathic practitioner who can tailor treatment for your specific needs, including those of your male partner. A good place to start is <www.fertility.com.au>. If you're someone who would consider IVF or other technological fertility treatments, try appropriate natural therapies first and give them sufficient time to work as these methods have a much higher success rate than IVF for fertility problems, depending on the problem, and are also better for your health and that of your baby. If IVF is necessary then pre-conception health care will still improve your chances of a healthy pregnancy and baby.

CHAPTER 16

IF NOT THE PILL, THEN WHAT?

So, if the Pill is not as safe and effective as you have been led to believe, what can you rely on for contraception? Over the next few chapters we'll be looking at what the alternatives are, how to mix and match methods to best suit your needs and lifestyle, and how to understand and make the most of the much quoted, but often misunderstood, 'effectiveness rates'.

What do we mean by contraception?

Methods used to avoid pregnancy typically work by contraception, abortion or sterilisation.

'Contraception' refers to those methods that prevent the ovum and sperm from getting hooked up and resulting in a conception. 'Sterilisation' refers to those methods that suppress or destroy the natural reproductive processes, or pathways, within our bodies. It is similar to contraception, but usually more permanent and difficult to reverse. 'Abortion' refers to those methods that prevent a fertilised ovum from continuing to develop naturally, its cells then passing with your next period.

As far as these definitions and hormonal contraception are concerned you'll find them described in detail in Appendix 1.

Barrier methods

Belinda, a 22-year-old student, and her fiancé were getting married in a few months, and had decided to wait until then to have sex. Over her summer holidays Belinda spent time researching contraception. After reading many pamphlets and articles online, and visiting a gynaecologist, she decided to stick to condoms. Why? 'Because, unlike the Pill, condoms won't mess with my hormones,' says Belinda. 'Later we can also look into fertility awareness so we won't have to use condoms so much,' she adds.

Barrier methods physically prevent sperm from reaching an egg, or ovum. These include condoms, diaphragms, cervical caps and female condoms. These are generally made of rubber although plastic versions are available if you find you're allergic to the rubber.

Whether rubber or plastic there are lots of different brands and styles of condom around. You may like to buy up a selection in different colours, tastes, scents and sizes, with or without lubricant or spermicide. You can try them out with your partner and give them a rating, or share them out with your friends and report back to each other.

While diaphragms and cervical caps need an experienced doctor or nurse to help you get the right fit, they can then be purchased in pharmacies and may last for up to two years. If you're allergic to rubber and need a plastic diaphragm you'll need to speak with the health practitioner fitting you. As plastic diaphragms are not widely available you may need to order one online after you're clear what size you need.

Both diaphragms and caps fit over the cervix preventing sperm from swimming up into the cervix, uterus and Fallopian tubes. Sperm left in the acidic vaginal environment die within a few hours, much more quickly than in the more nourishing environment of a fertile cervix, uterus and Fallopian tube. You need to check a diaphragm or cap regularly for holes or perishing and follow the instructions for washing and storing it.

My mum encouraged me to get a diaphragm instead of going on the Pill. At first I was put off by the idea of getting it fitted. But she pointed out it's not much different to using a tampon so I gave it a go—I'm so glad now! It doesn't interfere with sex and the rest of the time I'm not worrying about messing with nature.

ODELIA, 20

Cervical caps are generally less commonly used than diaphragms or condoms and require somewhat more skill for the user to fit, but once you're confident, these are as effective as diaphragms, and you may prefer their smaller size.

Condoms—rubber ones, at least—are widely available in pharmacies, supermarkets, and many public toilets—mostly men's—and don't require any input from a health professional. If you're a novice do read the instructions carefully for advice on how to fit, and when to remove, a condom. Plastic condoms are not often found in local pharmacies but can easily be ordered on the Internet. Enthusiasts prefer plastic to rubber not only because they're non-allergenic but also because they're significantly thinner and looser, being held in place by a ring at the base of the penis, and are said to offer a more 'natural' feel.

Female condoms are a more recent form of condom that fits inside the vagina and over the vulva, collecting sperm and preventing infection. An inner and outer ring keep the female condom in place. It may be a preferable option in some relationship situations and, although not widely available in pharmacies, can easily be ordered online.

The beauty of all barrier methods is that you use them when you need them and are free of them when you don't. As barrier methods work by preventing sperm and egg from meeting, they're a contraceptive method only and won't interfere with your overall fertility. And contrary to common perceptions, barrier methods can be very effective. Condoms used properly—and on *every* occasion of sexual intercourse—can be 98 per cent effective or more.[1]

Keeping free of sexually transmitted disease

Sex is the most physically intimate activity between human beings, other than pregnancy and birth. Because of this the opportunity for sharing the particular viruses, bacteria and parasites that love our warm, dark, moist places is high. These include chlamydia, herpes, gonorrhoea, and HIV, among many others. Condoms are, of course, essential for protecting yourself against sexually transmitted diseases when you're sexually involved with a potentially infected partner. In this context potentially infected means *not proven to be not-infected*. Male and female condoms are equally effective in preventing infection.

If you've noticed something different going on around your genitals or your mouth—like an itch, or lumps like pimples or warts, or an unusual discharge—do visit your doctor and get treatment. If you just want to be sure that you and your partner are disease free before you dispense with the condoms, your doctor will be able to test you both and let you know if you're all clear. If neither of you has been with another partner sexually, including oral or anal sex, then you can safely assume you're both disease free.

After an unpleasant experience with genital warts and crabs, Sally really understood the need for protection, at least until she had a steady boyfriend. While these problems weren't too hard to clear up she found they were a hassle and certainly unpleasant, far more so than the little inconvenience of using condoms.

Spermicides

Spermicides are chemicals—manufactured or naturally occurring—which kill or disable sperm, thereby preventing them from swimming up into the uterus and Fallopian tubes to fertilise an egg. Spermicides can be used alone but are more effective when used with another method, such as a condom, cap or diaphragm. Commercial spermicides come in many different forms—foam, gel, film and suppositories—and can be purchased over the counter in pharmacies or online. Most spermicides currently available contain either nonoxynol-9 or octoxynol, chemicals that disable sperm by removing the cell membrane.

To be effective, the spermicide must be placed deep in the vagina close to the cervix before sex. Creams, gels and foams can be inserted into the vagina using an applicator, or applied to a diaphragm, cap or sponge before their insertion. Other types of spermicides include vaginal contraceptive film, a thin sheet placed in the back of the vagina by hand, and vaginal suppositories.

Some spermicides offer protection right away but most need to be in the vagina at least fifteen minutes before sex so they have enough time to dissolve and spread. All forms of spermicides are only effective for one hour after insertion. Another application of spermicide is needed if more than one hour passes before sex, as well as before repeated sex. Don't wash out your vagina, or douche, for at least six hours after sex with spermicide use. (Not that your vagina needs to be washed out—it has its own marvellous inbuilt self-cleansing mechanisms.)

After an unhappy experience with an IUD—heavy, painful periods, and then a pregnancy—Louise was fitted with a diaphragm. She also purchased spermicide to use with it for extra protection. When she and her boyfriend Jake used it for the first time they fell about laughing as Louise, then Jake, tried to squeeze the slippery diaphragm into a long oval to slip up her vagina and into place. Now, many occasions later, Louise is happy with her diaphragm and slides it into place in a jiffy.

Due to its germicidal properties chemical spermicide can also kill the friendly bacteria that are essential for the healthy state of your vagina. This can cause vaginal irritation or bacterial imbalance, which may lead to thrush, especially if you use spermicide frequently, like every day. Spermicides may also irritate the surrounding skin or trigger recurrent urinary tract infections for the same reasons. Some men may also find commercial spermicides have an unpleasant effect on their penis.

Recent research has found vanadium, an organic metal compound, inactivates sperm more quickly than current commercial spermicide and also works at lower concentrations. When this becomes commercially available it may help you to avoid the problems that can accompany repeated use of current spermicides.

If you're into self-help and don't need fancy packaging, you may like to try some homemade spermicides. Russian research into fizzing Vitamin C tablets inserted into the vagina ten minutes before sex found this to be a reasonably effective spermicide. Lemon or lime juice can also be very effective. Professor Short and his team found that a 20 per cent concentration of lemon or lime juice in human semen irreversibly immobilised *100 per cent* of sperm in less than 30 seconds. Since the average volume of a normal human ejaculate is 2–6 millilitres then in order to guarantee at least a 20 per cent final concentration of juice it's recommend that 3 millilitres or a teaspoonful needs to be introduced into the vagina. To do this you may like to try using lemon juice to saturate a piece of sea sponge or a small ball of cotton wool—perhaps encased in muslin and knotted for easy removal—and placing this high in your vagina, taking care not to squeeze the juice out during insertion. Or, you may like to try one of the following lemon juice spermicide recipes.[2]

Lemon Juice Spermicide 1

Mix together 1 tablespoon of pure aloe vera to 1 teaspoon of lemon juice. If you're using aloe vera plant peel the skin and discard. Mash or blend flesh thoroughly to remove any lumps.

Lemon Juice Spermicide 2

1 cup water
$2\frac{1}{2}$ tablespoons cornflour (cornstarch)
1 teaspoon lemon juice
5 teaspoons salt
$2\frac{1}{2}$ tablespoons glycerine

Boil the water, add the cornflour and stir until it gels. Add the remaining ingredients and stir until combined.

Keep your Lemon Spermicide (either recipe) in a refrigerator in a sealed container and it will stay fresh and be effective for one week.

Spermicides are most often used with a barrier method to increase the effectiveness of both methods and you'll find that some brands of condom are already impregnated with spermicide. As we've already mentioned, some men and women find that they're allergic to commercially available spermicides. If this is the case with you, a home-made spermicide may be friendlier to your delicate genital skin.

Intrauterine devices (IUDs)

Inserting one thing or another into the uterus as a way to prevent pregnancy has been practised for millennia. Current IUDs are either inert and work by irritation, or they release copper or synthetic hormones into your body. The copper-releasing IUD is known as Cu-IUD and the synthetic progesterone-releasing IUD is known as LNG-IUD or IUS.[3]

At seventeen Julia went on the Pill for contraceptive purposes. A year and a half later she spoke with her gynaecologist about alternatives, as she'd found she didn't feel so good in herself while she was on the Pill. He suggested an IUD so Julia had one inserted. While she did experience heavier periods, which were painful for the first time in her life, the rest of the time everything was fine, and Julia felt the IUD was certainly an improvement on the Pill.

All types of IUD work contraceptively, in part by their effect on the lining of your uterus, and uterine and tubal fluid, as your body reacts to the presence of an irritating foreign body. The copper in the Cu-IUDs increases the foreign body effect which leads to a cascade of biochemical changes in the uterine lining, affecting local enzyme systems and hormone receptors. Copper ions from the Cu-IUDs are toxic to both sperm and fertilised ovum.

IUDs containing synthetic progesterone work via a combination of the IUD effect and the progesterone-only, or mini-Pill. The progesterone in these IUDs releases the hormone locally, and consequently a smaller amount reaches the rest of your body than if you were taking the mini-Pill, equivalent to about two mini-Pills per week.[4]

Inert IUDs are those which release neither hormones nor copper ions. These are no longer available in many countries and the Cu-IUD and LNG-IUD are more commonly used these days. It's estimated by the World Health Organization that 156 million women are currently using IUDs worldwide and of these 60 million are in China alone.

IUDs were much more popular until the severe illness and deaths caused by the Dalkon Shield™ in the mid-1970s. While advocates reassure women the IUDs available today are different and safer, pelvic inflammatory disease, ectopic pregnancy, increased bleeding and pain, expulsion of the device or loss of the 'string', incorrect insertion or perforation of the uterus during insertion are still of concern.

I got an IUD because I just didn't want to take the Pill anymore. It was easy in that I could forget about contraception, however I started to have bad go-to-bed cramps every month, and then after eighteen months I got pregnant anyway.

IRENA, 30

If you decide to try an IUD make sure the doctor you're seeing is well trained and experienced in IUD insertion to ensure correct positioning and timing of insertion. About 5 per cent of inert or copper IUD users have the device removed because of bleeding and pain within the first twelve months, and of the remainder about half report annoying bleeding.[5] And it's estimated that one in five women who have LNG-IUDs inserted have them removed within the first year.[6] IUDs work by both preventing egg and sperm from meeting and preventing the implantation of a fertilised ovum.

Sterilisation

Many couples who have completed their families opt for surgical sterilisation, either male or female. While male sterilisation, or vasectomy, is less invasive than female sterilisation, or tubal ligation, both still carry the usual risks of surgical procedures and depend on the skill of the surgeon. However, even with these procedures there is still a slight risk of pregnancy as tubes sometimes grow back together or the necessary waiting period after a vasectomy is not understood properly.

Sterilisation for women involves blocking or cutting the Fallopian tubes to prevent eggs and sperm from meeting and is performed while you're under a general anaesthetic. Once the surgery has occurred, female sterilisation is permanent. If you have this operation and change your mind later on, you'll need to use IVF techniques for a chance at having a baby.

Male sterilisation involves tying and cutting, or blocking, both vas deferens, or sperm ducts, to prevent sperm formed in the testes entering the ejaculate. While a vasectomy is somewhat easier to reverse than a tubal ligation, it nonetheless requires highly skilled micro-surgery to reconnect the vas deferens if a child is desired. Even then the chances of a pregnancy diminish about 10 per cent for each year since the vasectomy.[7]

As with all other methods of contraception, the side-effects of both male and female sterilisation need to be carefully researched and considered. These aren't always fully explained, or even known, by doctors performing these procedures.

Vasectomy has been found to increase the risk of cardiovascular disease, thyroid and joint disorders, cancer of the prostate, testicles and lung, diabetes[8] and dementia.[9] There is an increased risk of sperm granulomas, where sperm form knotty lumps around half a centimetre in diameter. They can cause pain like a kidney spasm and last for up to a year. And with tubal ligation, progesterone production often decreases in subsequent years leading to PMT, heavier periods, fibroids, premature menopause and depression. As an invasive surgery tubal ligation carries a risk of damage to nearby organs.[10]

The intra vas device

Still being trialled and considered promising is the intra vas device. This is a small plug of silicone gel which is used to block the vas deferens that connect the testicles and penis—effectively preventing sperm from being present in semen at ejaculation. The intra vas device could offer an alternative to surgical vasectomy and it is hoped that it will be more easily reversible. However, there is concern that this device might lead to a build-up of pressure behind the plug and damage the sperm production glands in the testes.

So far a pilot study of 30 men fitted with intra vas devices found that they had either no sperm in their semen or too few to be capable of conceiving. Further trials are underway with no general release date for these devices as yet available.[11]

It's yet to be revealed whether the intra vas device is a contraception or sterilisation method, or a method with elements of both.

Withdrawal

Withdrawal, also known as *coitus interruptus*, involves the withdrawal of your partner's penis from your vagina before he ejaculates, in this way preventing sperm from entering your reproductive tract. Its effectiveness depends in part on his skill at assessing 'time to ejaculation' and timely withdrawal, and also whether or not sperm enters his pre-ejaculate fluids—over which he has no control.

Withdrawal has historically been the method of choice in many parts of the world and was often practised as a form of machismo and chivalry.[12] Although it has suffered a poor reputation since mass-manufactured contraceptive methods have been around, withdrawal is known to be far better than nothing and has been responsible for reasonable success in preventing unwanted pregnancy. In Eastern Europe after the Second World War withdrawal was the main method of contraception used and resulted in some of the lowest birth rates in history.

Dr John Guillebaud, contraception expert and professor of Family Planning and Reproductive Health at University College, London, says of withdrawal: 'while encouraging the use of more modern methods, we should remember that—for many—this one works, and that it is a very great deal better than nothing in an emergency'.[13] In this sense the beauty of withdrawal is that it's always available and is completely free—certainly worth remembering as a backup.

We sometimes use withdrawal when I'm in the possibly fertile stage of my cycle, but we always avoid the definitely fertile times!

VIVA, 29

Similar to withdrawal, *coitus reservatus* involves your partner holding back ejaculation, either forgoing orgasm or enjoying orgasm without ejaculation. This method requires greater skill and body awareness than withdrawal. Nonetheless it has an illustrious heritage, having been practised by men in Indian and Chinese civilisations for thousands of years.

CHAPTER 17

WHAT ARE NATURAL CONTRACEPTION METHODS?

Within our drive for sexual intimacy are the powerful forces of fertility—Nature making sure of the continuation of our species with its rich diversity. With over six and a half billion human beings already on the planet, and counting, we could consider ourselves to be very successful at reproduction. This in itself is, of course, presenting its own problems. Now, as always, controlling our fertility is important for us as individuals as well as for society generally. There are basically two approaches to this. One is to switch off our fertility, either temporarily or permanently. The other is to understand it and work with that knowledge to our desired ends.

A similar approach to the former can be found in large-scale, broad-acre farming in which chemicals are used to destroy life forms that are not wanted—weeds and pests—and to promote those that are. The result of these methods, over time, is that the soil becomes seriously depleted and cannot produce anything without more and more chemical input. We know that food produced this way contains residues toxic to human beings and offers reduced nutrition and life force.

Representing the latter approach are organic, biodynamic and permaculture methods. These seek to understand fertility and life forces, and work with them productively. Using knowledge and intuition to work with land, soil, plants, animals, seasons and celestial cycles results in a rich, biologically alive soil, vibrant nutritious foods, healthy, happy animals and a diverse ecosystem. Food produced *this* way is packed with nutrition.

Natural methods of contraception, especially fertility awareness methods, represent this latter approach. Fertility awareness is a life skill gained when you become intimately familiar with your unique cycle of ovulation and menstruation. These methods can then be the basis from which you can choose the best method of contraception to use *when you're fertile*. This may be barrier, barrier with spermicide, non-genital-to-genital sexual practices or abstinence. While men are fertile all the time, unless they have fertility problems, women are not. So, once you know your fertile and infertile times, and allowing for safety margins, you may only need to use contraception one week in four, if your cycle is of average length.

The essential ingredients for successful natural contraception are a healthy curiosity about and friendliness towards your body, an understanding of how your body works, and a clear month-by-month choice about contraception. Not essential, but ideal, is cooperation between partners. The great secret of these methods is that, once learnt, they become automatic and then there's very little to do. You may revisit the learning process at times of change or to refresh your understanding, like after giving birth or a period of celibacy, but otherwise the knowledge you've gained becomes something you just know about yourself.

Discovering things about my body and how it works has been great. For my husband and I it's given us sexual freedom without all the negative side-effects.

ADRIENNE, 28

Many women have found that the real value in learning natural methods has been in gaining a deep awareness of themselves and their cyclical life. The usefulness of these methods as they relate to contraception then becomes a handy by-product. For Bea, 'it's great to be working with and nurturing my femininity and fertility instead of controlling it at all costs—to be treating fertility as a life-giving process and not some form of chronic or fatal disease'. And Rita has noticed, 'since I began charting my cycle it's been a real voyage of discovery around myself—an exhilarating experience like unlocking a secret code that I've carried inside of me all along'.

Natural methods of contraception are those that are device- and chemical-free and rely on an understanding of the processes and changing physical symptoms of fertility. As such natural methods aren't dependent on ongoing medical consultations—once learnt you can use them anywhere, anytime. That said, in these technological times certain equipment may be used to assist the learning or practising of some of these methods—equipment like thermometers, microscopes, ovulation testers, computers or calculators. However, these are optional and not intrinsic to using natural methods, except perhaps in the case of a thermometer when you practise the temperature method.

Natural methods hinge on an understanding of the viable life-span of sperm and eggs and that women are not fertile all the time. As your hormone levels change through your cycle, so do many of your bodily symptoms. Some of these are both easy for you to detect and precise in their indication of whether you are at a fertile or infertile time in your cycle. By pinpointing when these times of the month occur, you can, with your partner, plan and explore your sexual intimacy accordingly.

Another benefit of natural methods is that because they rely on understanding your fertility and using that knowledge to avoid conception, they're *fertility friendly*. That is, these methods pose no risk to your fertility and when the time comes that you do want to conceive, you will already be intimately familiar with the most likely time that conception could take place.

My partner thought it was a great idea—it seemed very common sense to him.
Using fertility awareness has given him more of an understanding of my
fertility as well.

JOY, 31

Rhythm method

One of the oldest methods of natural contraception is the rhythm method, in which expected ovulation is calculated from the length of your cycle for the preceding twelve months. Unprotected intercourse is then avoided during the time of expected ovulation, with generous margins for variations in the length of your cycle and for sperm life. The remainder of the cycle is considered 'safe'. The rhythm method relies on the fact that the second half of a cycle from ovulation to menstruation is close to a standard fourteen days, no matter what the total length of your cycle. However, this method works best if you have very regular cycles. Even then it can be hard to know when a regular cycle may change to an irregular one, as your menstrual cycle can be thrown out of kilter by many life circumstances, like travel, ill health or stress. These days when the rhythm method is used it is most often for backup information as the more precise fertility awareness methods offer far greater flexibility and effectiveness.

You may have heard the rhythm method referred to as 'periodic abstinence' as it has most often been used by Catholic couples practising abstinence during fertile, or possibly fertile, times of the month. Abstinence isn't necessary, however, for couples who aren't concerned with religious injunctions against using contraceptives, and condoms or diaphragms can be used at these times instead.

Of the two ways of identifying ovulation and its approach—by calculation or observation of body symptoms—observation has clear advantages. Most importantly it's more accurate than calculation, therefore less abstinence or protection is required at fertile, or possibly fertile, times for contraceptive purposes. And observation encourages involvement in, and awareness of, your reproductive processes, leading to even greater accuracy.

Fertility awareness methods

Fertility awareness methods include all those that teach you to read your body symptoms so that you can know, day by day, when you're fertile and when you're not. These include the Billings Ovulation Method, the temperature method, the sympto-thermal method and Natural Fertility Management as well as others using the same methods under different banners.

The Billings Ovulation Method

The Billings Ovulation Method, sometimes called the ovulation method, is named after Doctors Evelyn and John Billing, a husband and wife team who studied the cervical mucus changes as found at the mouth of the vagina. A healthy woman taught to read these changes can accurately predict when her mid-cycle ovulation will occur, plan a safe lead-up to this time, and know when her egg is no longer viable afterwards.

This method is so straightforward and obvious to women, once they've learnt to detect the variations in their own cervical mucus, that it has been used successfully by millions of women around the world, even those who have had no formal education. A World Health Organization survey in five countries showed that 95 per cent of women were able to return an interpretable chart of the changes in their cervical mucus by the end of their first cycle.[1] And studies have found that women taught to use the ovulation method correctly have a 98–99 per cent effectiveness rate.

Of all the ways available to you for assessing fertility on the ovulation cycle, observation of the changes in the cervical mucus is the most reliable and important.
FRANCESCA NAISH

Inside the cervix, the neck of the uterus, there are special cells in the hundred or so gland-like crypts. These constantly produce mucus, which changes in quantity and quality throughout the menstrual cycle, relative to the levels of hormones present. Low oestrogen, at the beginning and end of the cycle, results in scant amounts of sticky or tacky opaque mucus. As the levels of oestrogen rise and ovulation approaches, the mucus becomes more profuse, thinner, wetter and clearer. When oestrogen levels peak just before ovulation, the mucus is still wet to touch, becomes jelly-like and can be stretched between the fingers like raw egg-white. After ovulation, when oestrogen drops and progesterone increases, the mucus quickly becomes scant and tacky again.

To check your mucus, the easiest way is to collect some on your fingertips at the mouth of your vagina when you visit the toilet and before you urinate. You can then check it for quality and quantity and, while you're in the learning phase, record these observations at the end of each day.

When you record the colour, amount and texture of your cervical mucus, you will be amazed at how quickly a recognisable pattern emerges on your charts. After a while, the routine becomes automatic and requires little thought, and you'll find differentiating the various kinds of mucus very easy. Eventually you won't need to record your observations as you'll know clearly from your mucus where you are in your cycle. Of all the ways available to you for assessing fertility on the ovulation cycle, observation of the changes in the mucus is the most reliable and important.

When Robyn started to chart her body symptoms she found that 'my cycle turned out to be such a regular, straightforward one that I was amazed it hadn't always been obvious to me'. When Geraldine had her first appointment with a fertility awareness counsellor she was so relieved that she cried all the way home. 'I felt like I could now have my body back and functioning naturally instead of needing to use drugs and invasive devices,' she says.

Natural methods of fertility management give the power back to the individual. They enable you to deal with your fertility in a manner appropriate to each set of circumstances, instead of relying on second-hand, poorly explained and partial answers that encourage dependence on devices, chemicals and specialists.

FRANCESCA NAISH

The temperature method

The temperature method relies on the fact that your temperature is higher in the second half of your cycle, after ovulation, due to raised progesterone levels. Temperature readings, although they don't warn of an approaching ovulation like mucus observations do, can still be extremely useful. This is particularly true while you're learning fertility awareness.

Temperature is also an ideal backup if there are times when your mucus observations are confusing—for instance, if you have an infection. You can confirm through checking your temperature graph whether or not ovulation has occurred, and if you have entered the post-ovulatory infertile phase of your cycle.

To use this method you simply take your oral temperature upon waking, before doing anything else and at the same time of day, as far as possible. You then record your temperature reading on a graph. If there is some reason for a disturbance in your temperature—perhaps you woke late or have a fever—still record your waking temperature and make a note of the circumstances. You can adjust for the disturbance when you read your graph later.

In a classic graph, the temperature jogs along with small changes in the first half, or pre-ovulatory phase, of your cycle. It drops slightly just before ovulation and then, due to increased progesterone levels, rises by up to half a degree Celsius, or one degree Fahrenheit. It then stays up until just before, or during, your period, when it falls again. The most likely day for ovulation is the day of the temperature reading at the beginning of the rise.

With a little experience temperature graphs are easy to interpret at a glance. Temperature changes help to confirm that ovulation did, in fact, take place and are one of the most accurate ways of telling *when* it occurred. Knowing the most likely day for ovulation helps confirm for you the length of the post-ovulatory second half of your cycle. The effectiveness rate for the temperature method alone, when used correctly, has been assessed at 99 per cent.

You can learn to distinguish these marvellous and unmistakable signs that your body gives you and use this information to avoid or achieve conception, depending on your choice, for the whole of your fertile life.

FRANCESCA NAISH

More commonly, however, the temperature method is learnt in conjunction with the ovulation method, as well as other secondary symptoms. Temperature observations speed up recognition of the mucus patterns and confidence in using natural methods can happen much more quickly. You can then, if you wish, discard temperature readings as a regular part of your fertility awareness, relying instead on mucus observations. It's always useful, however, to have an understanding of temperature readings for times when your mucus observations may not be so reliable.

Janet's boyfriend suggested they try fertility awareness for contraception and while she liked the sound of the methods Janet wondered, 'Can I really get to know what's happening in my body well enough to rely on it for contraception?'. She decided to give it a go and soon found she loved filling in her chart every day. 'It was like doing a jigsaw puzzle and watching this amazing picture emerge,' Janet discovered. 'After fifteen years of cycling it was suddenly all clear to me,' she says. 'I quickly felt confident using this awareness as the basis on which to know when I was fertile and when I wasn't.' Twenty years later Janet reflects, 'I still feel this was one of the best things I ever did for myself.'

The sympto-thermal method

The sympto-thermal method incorporates both the cervical mucus and temperature methods, as well as observation of other body symptoms, or secondary symptoms, that fluctuate with the cycle, like the texture and position of the cervix. While the ovulation and temperature methods can be used on their own, employing both of these and observing secondary symptoms as well offers you greater clarification and confirmation of your fertile and infertile times. This also gives you more flexibility if any of your symptoms are unreliable for a time, like when you have a fever or your mucus pattern changes after giving birth.

Because fertility awareness and abstinence at fertile times are the only methods of contraception currently approved by the Catholic Church, a number of organisations that teach natural methods are Catholic Church approved or backed, as is the case with the Billings Ovulation Method and Natural Family Planning. The Justisse Method, the fertility awareness method (as taught by Ilene Richman) and Natural Fertility Management among others, on the other hand, are secular and health- and knowledge-based. These offer you and your partner flexibility and wellbeing in your sexual and reproductive choices, without religious injunctions, if this is your preference.

My cycle turned out to be such a regular, straightforward one that I was amazed that it hadn't always been obvious to me.

ROBYN, 36

The Justisse Method

The Justisse Method was developed by Geraldine Matus, a midwife and psychotherapist, in 1978 and is a combination of fertility awareness methods. Geraldine uses the term 'body literacy' and teaches this as a basis for reproductive choice and a healthy awareness of the menstrual cycle. She also considers this an important aspect of psychological, as well as physical, wellbeing for women. Geraldine is based in Edmonton, Canada.

Fertility awareness method

While this term can apply generically to all these methods, it's used here by Ilene Richman at the Fertility Awareness Center in New York to describe her teaching of fertility awareness, especially the three fertility signals of mucus, temperature and texture and position of the cervix. Ilene says fertility awareness can be used for pregnancy prevention, pregnancy achievement, insight into health, and for general empowerment and self-knowledge.

She also heads the Fertility Awareness Network, a coalition of fertility awareness instructors who operate mainly in North America but also in other English-speaking countries.

Natural Fertility Management

Natural Fertility Management is a unique combination of methods pioneered by Francesca Naish in the mid-1970s. She is a naturopath and author who specialises in reproductive health care at her clinic in Sydney, Australia. In Natural Fertility Management Francesca has combined the fertility awareness methods of mucus, temperature and the secondary signs of fertility with research into spontaneous ovulation. The result is a method that offers perhaps the most comprehensive understanding of our fertile and infertile times.

Knowledge is power. The more you understand what you are doing, and why, the more control you have.

FRANCESCA NAISH

Research into spontaneous ovulation, involving over ten thousand women, found that women sometimes ovulate outside their mid-cycle ovulation, potentially ovulating twice a month. While most conceptions do occur at mid-cycle, a second ovulation is possible; it is usually triggered by sexual stimulation and can result in a pregnancy. It was found that the times when a second ovulation may occur are predictable and that they can be calculated in advance. These times relate to the return every lunar month of the particular angle between the sun and moon that was occurring when you were born. These days it's very easy to calculate this for years ahead with tailormade software.

Naish has found that by adding an understanding of when a spontaneous ovulation may occur to the fertility awareness methods, this offers women an extra edge of success. Correctly applied, Natural Fertility Management has the same success rate as the theoretical success rate for the Pill.

Fed up with the Pill Carrie looked for information on natural methods and for a while could only get scanty and half-hearted instruction, mostly from doctors who, she says, 'seemed unsure and reluctant to give information on them'. This was during the 1980s. When Carrie finally came across Natural Fertility Management she found 'all the fine print was covered'. She adds, 'I'm really grateful to have found NFM and I'm extremely confident with it'.

Francesca Naish has written a best-selling book on fertility awareness, *Natural Fertility*, which we highly recommend for anyone interested in natural methods of contraception. And, with Jane, she has produced *The Natural Fertility Management Contraception Kit*, which includes a copy of *Natural Fertility*, and is an excellent way for you to learn these methods step-by-step.

I've been using fertility awareness for over a year now and I must say with much pleasure. I feel much more in touch with my body and newly confident around my sexuality. It's great to know exactly when I can conceive and when I can't.

GABBIE, 24

Natural methods and effectiveness

Researchers who studied 900 women using the sympto-thermal method of contraception over a ten-year period recently reported their findings, which indicated that 'the sympto-thermal method of contraception was as effective as the Pill in preventing pregnancy'.[2]

In addition to the sympto-thermal method the Justisse Method, the fertility awareness (as taught by Ilene Richman) and Natural Fertility Management all include teaching on when and how to use other methods of contraception at fertile times, ensuring seamless use of these for highly effective fertility management.

Studies of natural methods over the years have found a clear difference between effectiveness rates when these methods are well taught and when they are not. If you'd like to use a fertility awareness method we recommend you take the time to learn it properly. A vague guess at a 'safe time' is obviously going to be a lot less effective than a clear understanding of your body symptoms. Once learnt you will have this knowledge and these methods for the rest of your fertile life and, apart from providing effective contraception, this intimacy with your body and cycles can greatly enhance your self-awareness and sexual confidence.

Compared to the Pill natural methods also have a high rate of user satisfaction and continuation of use. Studies indicate that as many as six out of ten women who start taking the Pill discontinue before the end of the first year, and most of those during the first six months,[3] whereas virtually all women who learn fertility awareness, especially through an accredited counsellor, course or materials, continue to use these methods for the remainder of their fertile lives. Once gained this knowledge can't be unlearned and women find that their understanding of their cycle and fertility continues to deepen over time.

Contact details for where and how you can confidently learn fertility awareness methods are in the Recommended Reading and Resources section at the end of this book.

Fertility awareness has helped me to have a more complete sense of who I am as a woman and a deep appreciation of my fertility, which is very empowering.

JANETTE, 29

Mixing and matching methods

Effectiveness rates of various contraceptive methods are enhanced when used in combination. Barrier methods are frequently combined with spermicides, and these are often used during a woman's fertile time by couples practising natural methods.

By combining natural and barrier methods 'user fatigue' can be avoided as a condom or diaphragm may only be needed for a few days a month.

When barrier methods are relied on solely for contraception effectiveness may be compromised when a couple becomes tired of using them and may guess at, or hope for, a 'safe' time. By learning fertility awareness you add to your options and deepen your understanding of when you're fertile and when you're not. It's easier then to enjoy safe, contraception-free sex, and save the rubber for when you really need it.

The beauty of natural methods

Ultimately, the beauty of natural methods is that, for many women, gaining an understanding of their cyclic changes is not only healthier but also far sexier and more positive for relationships. In fact it's likely that the more you understand about how your fertility works the more amazing the whole process and design will appear to you. Bettina discovered that 'the rewards of using this method have extended well

> The great secret of these methods is that once learnt they become automatic and then there's very little to do.

beyond feeling confident about contraception'. She's noticed that 'it's opened up a whole new understanding of my body and has given me great peace of mind'. Vivienne 'loves the heightened awareness' of her body and cycles and has found this has given her 'a new sense of self-respect and empowerment'.

In the next chapter we'll help you to find the right contraception for you—contraception that will give you the best effectiveness rate and most compatible method or methods for your lifestyle.

CHAPTER 18

HOW TO FIND THE BEST CONTRACEPTION FOR YOU

For most of your fertile life you're not wanting to make babies when you make love, so it's well worthwhile fully exploring your contraceptive options. This will contribute to the quality of your sexual experience and relationship as well as the effectiveness of the method you choose.

It's very likely that different methods of contraception will be appropriate for you at different times. When considering these you can think about how they work, their effect on your health, if any, their usefulness in different situations as well as their effectiveness rates. You may have found that contraception has generally been offered to you as a one-size-fits-all rather than with consideration of what's possible and preferable for you, and your partner, with the right support.

Several decades ago birth was often managed in a very mechanical way—leaving women confused, distressed and disconnected from this profound process. This has slowly changed as women have explored ways to prepare for birth, so as to be present, conscious and actively involved when labour begins. As part of this process many women nowadays have a birth plan.

In the heat of sex you may not be so focused on precautions, nor is this the best time for clear thinking but, like a birth plan, if you have a carefully thought through contraception plan it means the clear thinking has already taken place and you're free to enjoy the moment. So, in the same way that you become expert in an array of skills during your adult life—skills that then become more or less automatic, like driving a car or managing your finances—consider taking the same approach to your fertility and become your own contraception expert.

There are still occasional challenges, but I always feel that we're making decisions together when it comes to lovemaking, which makes our sex life incredibly fulfilling.

MEGHAN, 24

Making the most of your doctor's appointments

You may be surprised to know that the medical profession has only recently come to have a role in dispensing advice on, and the means of, contraception. Prior to the arrival of the Pill only a minority of doctors actively assisted women with contraception—and even then it was primarily by fitting diaphragms and other barrier and intrauterine devices. Contraception, even for married couples, was a moral hotbed that many doctors wanted to avoid.

Professor Shearman, who in 1962 established family planning training at the University of Sydney's Faculty of Medicine, believed that 'the medical profession did not feel comfortable with contraception until the Pill became available; before that, it was regarded as messy and unpleasant. The Pill was clean and scientific, and the medical profession felt happier about prescribing it for women.'[1]

One of the prime modalities of general practitioners these days is drug therapy and as such doctors clearly have a role in prescribing the Pill. If you're looking for information on a range of contraceptive options, however, not all doctors will have the full breadth of training or information you need.

The doctor was not supportive when I wanted to come off the Pill. I asked about diaphragms and he said, 'No, they're not really used anymore'. The Pill is the only contraceptive offered to me by doctors that I have seen.

JENNIFER, 25

Quite naturally, Family Planning health professionals are concerned about preventing unplanned pregnancy across the community. Their focus may not include whether an individual woman wishes to get to know her own body and make contraceptive choices accordingly. Because of this, approaches that promote gaining that knowledge, like fertility awareness, tend to be given little attention by those involved in 'big picture' contraceptive services.

For these reasons many women have struggled to get the information they need. In Jane's case her doctor simply told her, 'Really, the Pill is the only way to go'. Nicola's experience was more mixed. 'The doctors I saw initially were quite dismissive when I suggested the Pill might be causing some side-effects,' she observed. 'When I started experiencing nausea and sometimes vomiting every morning I was just told to eat dry biscuits for breakfast.' Then, she adds, 'One of the main reasons I decided to come off the Pill is because my present doctor is so helpful and supportive.'

As there are, quite obviously, consequences to all your contraceptive choices, getting relevant and factual information as you need it is crucial to the choices you make. So, when looking for a health practitioner to advise you about your contraceptive options, as well as to fit, supply or teach the method, find one that you feel heard by and who will work *with* you. It could be a naturopath or another health practitioner who specialises in fertility and women's health, or a doctor who has received special training in contraception. You can also research methods for yourself, through books and on the internet. Then, you can work in partnership with your health practitioner when and as you need to.

What is informed consent?

As with all our major health decisions it's important that you have all the information you need to make a truly informed choice. Julie's doctor encouraged her to go on the Pill 'despite a niggling feeling that it didn't make sense to control my body chemistry that way'. Michelle reflects, 'I feel like I was left totally in the dark. The only information I got was the leaflet in the Pill packet and the doctor saying it was safe. He said it would probably increase my breast size and clear up my pimples as well.'

Many women have regretted not being fully informed when they consented to the Pill, hormonal implants, injections or other procedures. Making sure you have all the relevant information about the risks, benefits and how to correctly use the contraception you have chosen can make all the difference to your experience.

Five ways to inform yourself

- Learn as much as you can about your body as a woman.
- Assume that your body's natural rhythms and processes are there for a reason.
- Research all healthcare alternatives and remember that ads, and top internet sites, are placed there by those who have the money to do so. This doesn't mean they necessarily have the best information.
- Pay attention to how you feel and follow your instincts.
- Consult knowledgeable, health-conscious women about how *they* manage their reproductive health.

Ideally your healthcare professional will seek to fully inform you about the nature of the drug or procedure that you're considering, offer you reasonable alternatives and discuss the risks, benefits and uncertainties with you. You can then decide to accept or reject the drugs or procedures with full awareness of the consequences either way. Anything short of this, to your satisfaction, is not really informed consent.[2]

> *I wish I'd known about my cycles when I was an adolescent. I could have enjoyed them as I have done for the last ten years. It's very empowering to have this knowledge and be able to use it in such an important area of a woman's life.*
>
> **JULIE, 36**

The reality is that informed consent can rarely be realised within the confines of the mostly brief consultations with healthcare providers. So, as well as shopping for a doctor or health practitioner you feel happy with, make a point of informing yourself. In the same way that you would research a big purchase or further professional training before going ahead with it, it's a good idea to research your contraceptive options. It's certainly much easier to be well informed and make conscious choices than deal with the fallout of bad choices and *then* look at your options. After all, you're likely to be making decisions about contraception for decades of your life.

The wellness continuum

In addition to sourcing information about contraception you may find it useful to consider where you're at with your health overall. The wellness continuum is a way of positioning ourselves in regard to our health practices, our level of wellness and our health goals. We have included a brief summary of the wellness continuum here.

As far as we know, the wellness continuum was originally presented to post-graduate students at an integrative medicine course at Swinburne University, Melbourne, in 2000, by Drs Craig Hassard, Avni Sali and David Wignall.

Where do you fit?

Serious illness
Disease is advanced and has poor prognosis.

Illness
You require medications daily.

Rundown
You are tired, moody and 'blah' much of the time. Laboratory tests are inconclusive. You regularly use over-the-counter medications, coffee, sugar, food and alcohol for energy or relief. You're feeling worse with age.

No obvious symptoms
Danger zone—you feel OK but it's a false sense of security. Habits and behaviour patterns have established the early stages of degenerative disease.

Protected
You awaken refreshed every day. You don't get sick often and recover quickly. Nourishing food and supplements strengthen your body and immune system; you get regular exercise, and eliminate toxins from food, water and air.

Restored
You have clarity of mind and abundant energy. Your body rejuvenates itself. You have freedom from age-related degenerative disorders.

Vitalised

You're at the peak of health. You get maximum enjoyment out of life. You live up to your genetic potential and can expect vitality well into your ninth and tenth decade.

According to the presenters of the wellness continuum, the majority of people in the community are in the 'rundown' or 'no obvious symptoms' categories. Where do you see yourself along the wellness continuum? Where would you like to be?

If you want to make some changes to improve your overall wellness, remember: small steps, with simple changes over time, can create significant improvements in lifestyle and wellbeing.

The wellness continuum for contraception

Now, if we consider the wellness continuum in the light of contraceptive choices, we may come up with something like this:

Serious illness

While it's not likely you're still fertile a pregnancy and birth would be very problematic for you and your baby. If you are fertile use any contraception you can to prevent a pregnancy.

Illness

A pregnancy is not a good idea as it would further strain your health. Use whatever contraception you can to avoid it, but be aware that hormonal contraception may be exacerbating your health problems.

Rundown

While it may seem that the Pill or other hormonal contraception may not be adding much to the load your body is already carrying, be aware that it's further stressing your body. If you would like to feel better you may be considering changes to your diet and lifestyle under the care of a skilled health practitioner. During this process changing to a non-chemical, non-invasive form of contraception will contribute to your recovery. Learning natural methods as a basis for your contraception will contribute to the process of tuning in to your body rhythms, feelings and innate wellbeing.

No obvious symptoms

The Pill or other chemical methods of contraception may seem convenient to you and you may not have obvious side-effects. If you're aware of side-effects you may be willing to put up with them for the convenience of contraception you don't have to think about. But you also may like to consider the long-term problems that this approach to your health will bring, remembering that it takes more work and effort to regain good health than to maintain it in the first place.

Protected

You may have spent time on the Pill in your early adult life as you tried to manage your sex-life responsibly. Over time you became aware of the negative effects this was having on you. It seemed difficult to find alternatives that were medically recognised as effective. While you continued your search you used a combination of barrier methods and spermicide. You may be toying with the idea of learning natural methods, or if you have already started you have found this to be a great journey of discovery and you wish you'd known about them much earlier in your fertile life.

Restored

You may have taken the Pill briefly but quickly knew it was not for you. You have sought out alternatives that are healthier, including understanding how to use barrier methods for maximum effect, and learning about your own fertility cycles to know when you are fertile and when you are not. This understanding has been a revelation and has further contributed to your understanding of yourself as a woman. Your level of health and connectedness to your own body allow you to enjoy a rich sexuality and relationship life.

Vitalised

You instinctually knew the Pill was not for you and have never taken it. It was an obvious step for you to learn about your own fertility cycles as a way to understand and manage your fertility. This is now simply part of what you know about yourself and contributes to the subtle sensitivity and enjoyment you have in your own body. As time goes on your experience of your fertility and cycles becomes more and more profound and deeply pleasurable. You feel vital and relaxed and this informs your instinctive healthy choices around sexuality and relationships.

How does your choice of contraception fit with where you see yourself on the wellness continuum?

Questions to ask yourself

Thinking about where you are in life's fertility-sexuality continuum, and where you may be heading next, is also a very useful way for you to assess what contraception is going to suit you. You may want to have a pen and paper handy to make notes as you read the next couple of pages.

Are you single and enjoying brief affairs? Are you single and looking for someone special? Do you have a boyfriend or lover but you're not necessarily monogamous? Are you in a steady relationship? Are you newly married but not planning children just yet? Are you considering starting a family in the next few years?

Do you have a young child and would like another sometime in the next few years? Have you probably completed your family? Have you most definitely completed your family?

Have you decided that you don't want any children? Are you pre-menopausal and probably not very fertile, but *really* don't want to conceive now?

Once you have determined where you are in the fertility continuum then ask yourself the following questions.

Do you need protection from STDs? How would you feel about an unplanned pregnancy? What would you want to do about an unplanned pregnancy?

What health risks or problems are you willing to put up with in order to have effective contraception that you don't have to think about? What efforts are you willing to make to have effective contraception without a risk to your health and that of your partner? Share these questions with your partner and see what he thinks.

Your answers will suggest certain forms or categories of contraception. As you consider these, along with your overall health goals, you may like to make a contraception plan.

Your contraception plan

If you've thought through all the issues in relation to your contraception and have a good plan, you're far more likely to be successful, as is the case with most things in life.

How would you rate your current contraception on a scale of one to five, with one being totally unhappy and five being totally happy. Are you confident about your use and understanding of your current contraception? Is your answer a two? A five? And what about your partner?

Next, consider backup contraception. If for some reason you couldn't use or rely on your current contraception what would you use as a backup? Out of five, how confident are you in using and understanding your backup contraception?

Along with your current and backup contraception, how many other forms of contraception do you have available or do you have experience with? Make a list of these.

Now, considering your contraceptive needs and health goals, is your current contraception, backup and contraceptive experience working well for you? If there's room for improvement consider what else is available and find out more about it. Adding skills and knowledge can only improve your overall experience of contraception. To help you think this through we've included a blank form, 'My Contraception Plan', in Appendix 5. You can also use this plan to help you think through your needs regarding STD protection.

Having learnt fertility awareness many years ago I know my cycles are really regular. However, if I'm really busy and feeling less in touch with my cycle I'll use an ovulation tester to be sure that I've ovulated.

MIRANDA, 37

In the next chapter we explain what success rates mean and show you how to make the most of them for your own contraceptive effectiveness.

CHAPTER 19

MAKING THE MOST OF SUCCESS RATES

So, you want the best guarantee possible that you won't get pregnant until you decide you're ready to. What do success rates *really* mean? And how do they relate to your choices about contraception?

A recent study found that a surprisingly large proportion of women become pregnant while using birth control, either because they used it incorrectly or because the methods were inappropriate for their lifestyle.[1] As we've already seen, millions of women get pregnant every year even while using the Pill or other hormonal contraception. But perhaps even more shocking is that, according to the World Health Organization, if every fertile couple on the planet used contraception perfectly all the time, there would still be six million unplanned pregnancies every year.[2]

While you may be powerfully motivated to use contraception with all possible care and awareness, and this will certainly give you the best chance of success, there's still no guarantee that pregnancy won't occur. This can be a big stress. However, if you're able to have open and honest conversations with your partner around this possibility, it can be a good way to share the concern and alleviate any anxiety you might be experiencing.

> *I worry about getting pregnant—it freaks me out. A baby is just not an option for now, so it's often hard for me to relax and enjoy sex.*
> **AMELIA, 20**

OK, so that's the bad news. The good news is that by having a thorough understanding of contraception and choosing a method or combination of methods that you're happy with and use consistently, you'll have the best possible chance of successful contraception. As an example of how this can work, family planning expert Dr John Guillebaud says careful condom users are known to do better than poor Pill users.[3]

When considering effectiveness rates, remember that these statistics are averaged from a whole lot of studies reflecting the experiences of tens, hundreds or thousands of women. An individual woman's success or failure with contraception may or may not represent the average. For yourself, success rates are part of the information you need so that you can decide about contraception but they are by no means the only factor to take into consideration. Understanding different methods in relation to your health, relationship, lifestyle and contraception balance will help you to discover *what will work best for you*. You may need to try out a number of types of contraception before you find one, or a mix, that you can settle with. While exploring take the best care you can by doubling up your protection.

Some tips on deciphering success rates

The success rates of methods of contraception are generally quoted in 'per hundred woman-years'. This means that if a method is quoted as

99 per cent effective then if one hundred fertile, sexually active women were to use the method for one year, one would get pregnant, on average. These odds may sound pretty good, but consider this: if these hundred women were to use the method for ten years, the equivalent of one thousand woman-years, then we would expect ten pregnancies. So, over a ten-year period the effectiveness rate would be 90 per cent: that is, if you used the method for ten years you would have a one in ten chance of a pregnancy during that time.

When considering success rates it's also important to note whether the rate quoted is a *theoretical success rate* or a *user success rate*. A theoretical rate relates to the best possible rate for this method if used perfectly at all times. The theoretical success rate accounts only for failures of the method itself.

A user success rate is the rate recorded by people actually using the method. Some may not have been taught to use a method correctly, while others may forget to take their Pill, lose their diaphragms, run out of condoms, take a known risk, have an illness or use a medication that interferes with their contraception. Any of these factors can diminish the effectiveness of the contraception, on top of failures that relate to the method itself.

The theoretical and user rates for a particular method can vary considerably, as we have seen with the Pill. If you're willing to tolerate the side-effects of a method which is offering you a theoretical success rate of 99 per cent, you may be less willing to do so when considering how that translates into a user success rate over an extended period of time.

Managing risk

Reversible contraceptive methods that offer the very highest success rates are generally those that are the most invasive and have the most serious side-effects, like an injection, an implant or a LNG-IUD. The appeal of these methods is that they don't rely on daily remembrance. However, when assessing the effectiveness of these methods we also need to consider that they have high drop-out rates, with about one in three women who receive implants and about one in five LNG-IUD users having them removed within the first year. All other methods that rely on remembering and correct use, either daily or at the time of sexual intercourse, will work to the best of their capacity—and nearer to their theoretical success rate—if you're happy with, and understand, the method.

Careful condom users are known to do better than poor Pill users.
DR JOHN GUILLEBAUD

When you're considering success rates as part of your decision-making process check out the rates supplied by manufacturers or method teachers, as well as those arrived at by independent research. Avoid as much as possible success rates offered to you as hearsay as these often become wildly distorted into fantasy 'perfect' success rates or horror failure rates. Especially be aware that the Pill is often presented as much more effective than it actually is and fertility awareness methods are often confused with the rhythm method and presented as having poor effectiveness when this isn't the case.

A girlfriend of mine got pregnant on the Pill—it was a big surprise to her, she thought it just shouldn't have happened.
DAVID, 27

The things to remember about contraception are that, first, no method of contraception is 100 per cent effective, including the Pill, implants, injections and sterilisation. Secondly, more important for effectiveness than relative success rates, as long as you're considering reasonably good methods to start with, is carefully choosing a method, or methods, that best suits you, your relationship, your lifestyle, your health goals and your stage of life. And finally, for maximum effectiveness of your chosen method, take the time to learn how to use it correctly and use it correctly on all occasions.

To be considered *highly effective* a method of contraception needs to have a failure rate of one per cent or less. However, if you're combining methods you can achieve this level of effectiveness with methods that on their own may not be 99 per cent effective but together *are* highly effective. Appropriate combinations of methods, like barriers with spermicides or barrier methods with fertility awareness at fertile times, will give you highly effective contraception.

The power of intention

The effectiveness of your contraception can be undermined by any mixed feelings you may have about it. It might be that you're on the Pill but worry about the effects it might be having on you. You might not want to look like you *planned* to have sex. You may not consciously want to conceive but you might fantasise about a 'mistake'. Or, you might worry about your capacity to conceive. Maybe you find yourself getting clucky when you fall in love or when friends are having babies. Any of these scenarios can lead to diminished care when using contraception. Or you may just be very busy and not altogether focused on contraception. Quite naturally, when sex happens you may be much more interested in the emotional intensity and pleasures of the moment than in being really precise about your contraception.

One simple way to address these potentially undermining factors is—with or without your partner—to make a clear intention at the beginning of each cycle *just for the duration of that cycle*. It's much easier to be clear about what you want in the short term. To do this: on the first day of your period, become aware of any factors that may undermine your use of contraception. Clarify your intention that you don't want to conceive during *this cycle*. You may like to use some of the quiet meditative space of menstruation to visualise using your chosen method(s) of contraception successfully.

We decided we both needed to take responsibility for contraception. For me understanding my cycles has made me appreciate my fertility and I feel more like a real woman. Our sex life is also better because of the awareness and creativity we've put into it.

REBECCA, 29

As you move towards embracing the fundamental connection between fertility and sexuality, you're more able to make healthy choices for yourself and about your relationships. And then, perhaps surprisingly, you may find this adds to your intimacy and sexual connection or, at the very least, serves to clarify what it is you want in a relationship.

In the following chapters we explore how cycles, and your menstrual cycle in particular, are important for your health, wellbeing and relationships.

CHAPTER 20

WHAT'S THE POINT OF A CYCLE?

To have a period or not to have period, that's the question. Is it OK to switch your periods off? Are cycles inherently important? Thinking about the bigger picture of cyclical life might not seem very relevant to your immediate desire for reliable contraception or healing your period problems, but appreciating the inherent logic and power of cycles for sustaining life—your body's and the planet's—might help you to get clearer on whether the Pill is really a good thing for you.

From the deep internal rhythms of our bodies to the great rhythms of Nature—the seasons, the moon, and the circling planets—cycles are influencing, regulating and touching all aspects of our lives. We're profoundly cyclical beings. When you're in touch with cyclical rhythm you feel more 'in the flow', as though you're connected to a bigger life force beyond your ordinary, everyday life.

A cycle is a system of generation and regeneration—of birth, growth, peaking, falling away and ending to be followed again by birth. It's a process of expansion and contraction, of activity and rest. What this means for you is that your body is in constant rhythmic change, much of which is happening beneath your awareness. In fact sameness is deadening, both physically and psychologically. It's your changing nature that's keeping you alive (literally), and lively, responsive and creative.

The true nature of health . . . is flux, flow, cycle and movement. Disease manifests where there is fixity.
ALASTAIR GRAY, HOMOEOPATH

On the Pill Meghan had suffered bad moods, hysterical crying bouts, anxiety and depression. At 22, she came off the Pill after taking it for two years. The experience was revelatory. 'The Pill,' she said, 'is a pattern but it's not your pattern.' Her extreme moods cleared up, and learning about her body through fertility awareness made her realise how much more in tune with her life she can be. At certain times of the month she knows she can expect certain things—when she's fertile and infertile and when her period is due—and knowing this puts other aspects of her life in context as well. For instance, knowing that she's fertile helps her understand why she feels so sexy and horny, joyous when she sees a newborn baby, and generally in a good mood. Knowing that her period is due helps her accept her feelings of ill ease with her body and a general edginess and anxiety. Connecting to the rhythm of her body has been really empowering: 'now that I'm off the Pill the mind/body continuum is really clear to me, I can feel the interactions, I'm grounded in myself'. Meghan is having the delicious experience of aliveness that naturally arises when you're feeling really good inside your own skin and connected to the rhythms of your cycle.

Cooperation not control

When we try to control nature and biology, rather than to understand and cooperate with them, there are always consequences.
DR CLAUDIA WELCH, AYURVEDIC PRACTITIONER

While your biology doesn't rule you, it's wise to cooperate—to develop a healthy relationship and routine with it, understanding and working with the flow. Like in any relationship, there's your own timing and the other person's timing. Sometimes these clash. You want to go ahead with something and someone else isn't ready. You can fight these tensions and try to force the issue. Or, you can learn to work with them. By facing the difficulties in your relationships, you can make them stronger, more creative and loving, and you grow too. You can learn to appreciate what others bring to an issue and learn more flexibility. The tensions can make you look at things in yourself that you might not like. Uncomfortable though this is, you can become wiser, smarter and more tolerant.

Similarly, it's wise to engage with your body's rhythm. That means there'll be times when you have lots of energy and drive, and times when all you want to do is chill out; times when you feel very sensitive and vulnerable, and times when you feel tough and could take on anything. This is entirely normal and healthy. When you cooperate with your body's rhythms you can feel so much more alive and present.

You've probably noticed how your feelings and energy levels can shift with the seasons. Spring is a time of newness and wanting to be out there again, leading to the high, easy time of summer. Autumn brings a shift in mood, drawing us inwards to the quiet and stillness of winter. And just as you accept the changes in your mood and lifestyle as the seasons change, so it's a good idea to flow with your inner bodily seasons.

As the Earth goes around the sun, our bodies change with those cycles. So we may feel like falling in love in spring or getting depressed in winter, and that's because the biochemistry of the body changes as the Earth transforms itself in these cycles.[1]

DEEPAK CHOPRA

At some point in your life, either through too much partying, insomnia, shiftwork or crossing time zones on a long haul flight, you'll have disturbed your circadian rhythm—that's your day/night rhythm—and thus know how disorienting and unproductive that can be. While from time to time you can cope with interruptions to this cycle, if it's continually disrupted this can be disastrous for your overall psychological and physical wellbeing. You can start to feel more and more irritable and reactive, and generally rundown. This can lead to depression or longer-term health problems from a poorly functioning immune system to an increased risk of cancer.[2] Interrupting your menstrual cycle will have similar consequences, although it might not show up immediately.

Taking the Pill is like damming a river—the water becomes stagnant.
LUKE, 30

How to stay on top of your game

To stay active and productive at work, with your friends and family, or at the gym, you need times of rest and retreat. To be creative we need times of simply daydreaming and letting go. There are times, of course, when we have to handle a lot of stress and activity, and this can be very stimulating. However, what makes stress stressful is when it doesn't let up and you don't have any sense of control over it.

Dr Ernest Rossi, an expert in the study of biological rhythms, researched 'ultradians', meaning rhythms taking place many times a day.[3] He found that we have an hour and a half cycle of activity and focus, followed by a twenty-minute drop in alertness and energy—that's the moment when you suddenly find yourself yawning, looking out the window or feeling like a break for a coffee and a snack. This cycle of alertness and loss of alertness is a natural built-in rhythm of

> Having a strong rhythm and routine in your life is fundamental to building a healthy and sustainable life.

activity and rest, and his recommendation is that we take the twenty-minute break. While it may not always be possible to down tools for twenty minutes, or to persuade your boss this is a good idea, a good yawn and stretch, getting a drink or going for a brief walkabout can refresh you.

When you fail to listen to the body's signals, according to Rossi, you start to lose your concentration, make mistakes, get cranky and have accidents. Continuing to ignore your need for a break can lead to more and more stress and eventually illness. He calls this the ultradian stress syndrome. However, when you cooperate with your body's natural ebb and flow you get the ultradian healing response—that good feeling of ease and wellbeing that naturally follows when you're tired and let yourself have the freedom to take well-deserved rest. The twenty-minute troughs, rather than being a waste of time, are vital windows of opportunity in the day for your body and psyche to rest, reorganise and reorient, improving your overall creativity and performance.

You are rhythm, you are made of flesh, blood, bones and rhythm. Rhythm is what keeps you alive . . . Things happen to knock us out of rhythm, but it is a more natural state to be in rhythm, to be in sync. Rhythm is a spiritual practice and a very inexpensive deep medicine.
MICKEY HART, DRUMMER FOR THE GRATEFUL DEAD

How often do you soldier on using unhealthy food, coffee or drugs to see you through while ignoring the 'downtime' signals from your body? Far from creating vitality, the constant hits are creating artificial highs that actually draw on your energy reserves. Like overusing your credit card when you don't have the income to match, it may feel great to spend up but the arrival of your credit card statement can be sickening.

Acupuncturist Jost Sauer in his book on addictions, *Higher and Higher*, outlines how constant 'hits' or artificial highs deplete your body and spirit. He also offers lots of great ways to build vitality and experience natural highs by cooperating with the body's cyclical systems.

Having a strong rhythm and routine in your life is fundamental to building a healthy and sustainable life—an exercise routine, healthy eating habits, sufficient sleep and times to chill and reflect. When this is more or less happening and you do have times of intense stress, you'll be able to cope as long as you come back to your routine afterwards. Sauer also recommends that we supplement our self-care program with support from such things as counselling, massage, acupuncture or naturopathic treatment.[4]

> To stay active and productive we need times of rest and retreat. To be creative we need times of daydreaming and letting go.

Vitality tips for that energy low at work

- Drink plenty of purified water, especially in that low energy moment in the afternoon.
- Eat a protein snack such as raw nuts, or a piece of cheese.
- Stop all work for five minutes—yawn, stretch, lay your head on your desk and close your eyes for a few minutes of micro napping.
- Tap lightly on your body—the top of your head, around your eyes, above and below your mouth, down your neck, your shoulders, lower back, around your stomach, even down your legs.

Boosting your creativity

Taking some chill-out time can be surprisingly creative too. Rossi notes certain historical figures like Leonardo da Vinci and Thomas Edison, who got their inspirations *after* they had dropped their focused activity.

Instead of pushing on, they took a break and out of that came their break-through idea. When you stop and chill for a moment, perhaps wander off to get yourself a drink, you may notice you get more perspective.

Your period is a similar window of opportunity. It's your natural renewal time that can give you breakthrough ideas about your life and any creative project you're involved in. However, to access that insight you do need to relax when you bleed, letting yourself be more dreamy and slow.

Cycles and your health

There's increasing scientific evidence that destruction of biological rhythms in general results in loss of health. Life rhythms increase stability, save energy and support efficiency within the organism.[5]

The abnormal development found in cancer cells may be connected to disturbances of rhythms. Cancer patients can have extremely reduced sleep quality indicating a disturbed circadian rhythm. Disturbance of biological rhythms is apparent in cancer cells and vessels supporting cancer. A circadian clock that's humming along as it should is increasingly being recognised as an important tumour suppressor.[6]

A recent development in medicine considers time of the day and stage of a woman's menstrual cycle so that drug therapy or surgery occurs at the optimum time. The time in her cycle when a breast cancer patient undergoes surgery can influence the success of her treatment.[7] And then there's that highly delicate operation called 'having your legs waxed'! You may have noticed that it's much more painful just before your period.

Many of your body's vital signs—neurological and endocrine functions, temperature fluctuations, hormone and enzyme production, electrolyte excretion and, of course, the sleep/wake cycle—are governed by the circadian rhythm, so it stands to reason that interruption of those natural rhythms will cost you.[8]

The high cost of ignoring nature's rhythms

Global warming is now alerting us to the enormous cost of ignoring the rhythms and processes of the natural world. Similarly, there are great problems in how we manage our farmland. In 2003 researchers at Essex University worked out that British taxpayers spend up to £2.3 *billion* every year repairing the damage that industrial farming does to the environment and human health.[9]

Traditionally, crops were rotated and fields allowed periods of fallowness—nature's equivalent of our 'downtime'—so that the soil could recover naturally. Today, fallowness looks like wasted resources, whereas it's an important part of an integrated system of caring for soil that maintains genuine vitality, as compared to artificially stimulated productivity that comes from inorganic petrochemical fertilisers.

Getting in sync with your menstrual rhythm

Just as you'd think someone was mad to suggest you ignore your circadian rhythm, it's equally mad to suggest you ignore or shut down your menstrual cycle. It's no less a cycle than any of the other cycles of life. We tamper with it at our peril.

In Ayurvedic terms you could say that the Pill replaces the body's natural intelligence with synthetic rhythm. Then, when women quit the Pill, the body's natural intelligence has atrophied and it takes a while to re-establish balance.
DR CLAUDIA WELCH, AYURVEDIC PRACTITIONER

When the menstrual cycle is interrupted through stress or taking the Pill, this will affect your emotional and physical wellbeing. Cooperating with the natural checks and balances of cyclical life in general, and for us women of our menstrual cycle, could prove in the long term the really cool, smart, wise thing to do if we want to get the very best out of life, and not stuff up the planet in the process.

Create your own menstrual dreaming chart to tap into your 'inner seasons'

In Appendix 6 you'll find a sample chart to help you create a menstrual dreaming chart of your own. Either draw one on your computer or do it by hand. Use A3 size paper if possible. Or you could photocopy and enlarge the chart in the appendix. Each segment of the chart is a day of your cycle. On the outermost rim of the segment write the day of the cycle—day one is the first day of bleeding—and in the inner rim the date.

At the end of each day, perhaps as part of your routine before climbing into bed, write a phrase or two that captures your feelings in the segment for that day such as: really productive, easy flowing, sexy and attractive, magical, inspired, pumping with ideas, lots of energy, anything's possible today, ordinary, ho hum, irritable, low, no focus, dreamy, lost. And include any standout events such as great sex, a fight with your friend or partner, a powerful dream (which would be worth recording in more detail in an accompanying journal), going wild with the credit card, winning the lottery! If you have an artistic bent you can draw as a way to record your experience.

Aim to do the charting for at least three cycles—or go for longer if you can—and notice the unfolding pattern of your inner seasons. Charting helps you to connect with yourself; it is grounding and confidence-building and can give you real understanding that can feel quite magical.

If you suffer with PMS or pain, the charting will give you insight into how to manage your life better and reduce stress, which in turn will reduce your symptoms.

At 34 Libby is a director of her own highly successful company and has been using the charting to manage her PMS and energy levels. Now that she knows when her period is due she's more accepting of it and has more patience with herself, particularly when she feels exhausted before bleeding. She's noticed times of high clarity and productivity tend to happen at certain times of the month. Now that she knows about her 'powertime' in the cycle, she leverages that for success. With her enormously pressured schedule, being more connected to her cycle is helping her to feel more grounded and mindful of taking care of herself as well as her business.

Clare, 22, found that getting in touch with her inner seasons helped to ease her period pain and also to handle all the 'stuff' going on in her life much more wisely. 'I can move through challenging situations and circumstances in a positive way without becoming negative towards myself.' Acceptance of her different moods has meant that she doesn't force herself to go out if she's feeling low or a bit tired; instead she enjoys being chilled and quiet and then feels much more peaceful in herself.

CHAPTER 21

HOW TO GET CONNECTED

There's nothing more wonderful than feeling comfortable in your own skin, at ease with the ebb and flow of things. Life hums, you have energy and it all feels effortless. You're connected. At such times even problems are less like 'problems' and more like creative opportunities or interesting challenges that you willingly embrace. Being in touch with the whole of you is the key to this greater harmony. Anything that shuts down a part of you, especially a cycle, needs a warning sign such as they have on the side of cigarette packets saying that this is hazardous for your health.

On the Pill Nessa felt numbed and totally disconnected from herself. Now that she's off it she's really loving being in touch with her own rhythms and cycles and knowing where she's at fertility-wise. Katie felt ripped off after being on the Pill for twenty years, cheated of her true feelings for all that time. Many women report similar experiences when they come off the Pill.

I feel like everything just flows now I'm off the Pill.
MICHELLE, 35

Rhythm and depression

A result of not being connected to rhythm is depression. The epidemic of depression in the West is happening for both women and men, and the highest rate of incidence is among 18- to 24-year-olds.[1] Disturbingly, the depression rate for girls doubles at puberty. Until puberty, the rates for girls and boys are the same, however, depression increases in females once the ovarian hormones surge and cycling begins. The highest incidence is reached between the ages of 22 and 45. After menopause, the rates of depression in men and women are the same once again.[2] A similar pattern shows up across many cultures.

Studies have found that negative attitudes to periods impact girls' and women's experience of their cycles and themselves. How you experience menarche—that's your very first period—can affect your feelings about yourself and your experience of menstruation. Menarche is a highly sensitive time. The messages you receive about yourself and your body at that time, whether positive or negative, can imprint on you quite deeply.

The value we place on menstruation has a direct correlation with the value we place on ourselves as women.[3]
LARA OWEN, TEACHER AND WRITER

If you have a daughter it's very important to make sure she receives unambiguous, affirming and gentle education about puberty in an environment in which she can safely ask any of those curly, embarrassing questions. Shushann Movsessian, psychotherapist and teacher on puberty for over fifteen years, has written an excellent book for girls called *Puberty Girl*, approaching the issues with clarity, humour and real affirmation of girls' intelligence and strength. And as a mum you'll find Jane's book, *A Blessing Not a Curse*, full of useful tips and ideas. The following are a few key points you can consider at this time.

Tips for mums

- Think through your own experience of puberty and how you'd like it to be for your daughter.
- Talk with other women about their experiences.
- If you haven't already, get to know *your* cycle. Read, chart, write in a menstrual journal and simply *notice and observe*.

With your daughter:

- Be open all along about your periods, explaining in simple age-appropriate ways what's going on.
- As she starts to develop, talk about what's unfolding, look at books together, answer questions, find answers if you don't have them already.
- Talk about what to expect when her period comes—how to manage if it comes at school, when at a friend's house or on camp.
- Have a look at a range of menstrual pads together.

When her period arrives:

- Plan something special—keep in mind what would be comfortable for your daughter. This may be on the day of her first period, or around that time, or within the year.
- Offer her your heartfelt congratulations and a day at home with you. You may like to do some fun things together—like have a massage or a manicure, or run her an aromatherapy bath.
- You might make a special meal or her favourite cake, put beautiful flowers in her room, give her a piece of jewellery from your mother or grandmother or a special diary or other gift.
- Support the father's relationship with his daughter and the importance of their ongoing connection during her teenage years.

Losing one's rhythm is excruciating. It's worse than excruciating, it causes one to not recognise oneself on the inside, and not feel quite alive and then yearning for its return.

LUCY (AFTER BRAIN SURGERY), 39

Jessie's story

Jessie was your average budding girl—into horses, ballet and hanging out with her friends. She was confident, achieving well at school and optimistic about the future. When she was almost twelve years old and just before her first period, her parents' acrimonious separation hit her hard. Jessie went with her dad and her sister stayed with her mum. Soon after, on holiday with her father, she got her first period but was too scared to speak to him about it. She remembers being at the swimming pool, seeing the blood and experiencing her mind open up. 'All of a sudden I could see everything around me external of my mind. I saw Dad as human and having a life and Mum too. I saw all their issues and their hurt.'

She also started to have painful periods and heavy bleeding and was put on the Pill by her doctor. Soon after, her world seemed to collapse—in her second year of high school a black cloud descended engulfing all the positive aspects of herself. At eighteen she attempted suicide. 'I just wanted to go to sleep and never wake up,' she said. At nineteen she discovered alcohol and drugs, which gave her a temporary feeling of being happy and more normal. But at 22 she attempted suicide again and after this got professional support and went on antidepressants. At 39 antidepressants have been her support for most of her adult life. Occasionally she has tried stopping but has experienced that strange expanded vision that she had at the time of her first period. It's always felt too much and she didn't know any other way to block it out.

Jessie has never really understood why she was depressed since her childhood was pretty happy, apart from her parents break-up. But while

> While depression can have multiple causes, making sure a girl has a positive experience at her first period is a vital step in ensuring she grows up feeling good about herself and her life.

attending a workshop on preparing her daughter for puberty she heard how depression in girls can be connected to what happens to them at menarche. As she listened she felt the old familiar signals of her depression—sleepiness, heaviness and wanting to be swallowed up by the earth—come over her. Only when asked to share her story was she able to lift herself out of it. Then the penny dropped—this was what had happened to her. Tears welled up, tears of relief. In that highly sensitive, charged time of her first period she had been overwhelmed by her parents' divorce and their pain, and had no way to deal with it.

In that same workshop she learnt how during menstruation she could have a much more heightened awareness for sensing and knowing things. Suddenly she had an explanation for the intense visions she experienced. It was revelatory. She resolved then and there to come off the Pill and is now slowly weaning herself off antidepressants as well. Already she's feeling clearer and stronger and, most importantly, that she's not crazy for having these intense visionary experiences.

Creating your menarche celebration party

If you had a hard time when you went through your first period, or even if it was a non-event, there are things you can do to rectify this, which may help you to feel happier in yourself. Have a menarche celebration party with a small group of girlfriends you trust—probably no more than about four to keep it intimate. Prepare the space with flowers, candles, a photo of the younger you and any other significant objects, perhaps connected to the women of your family such as a special piece of jewellery. And bring some celebration food and drink to enjoy afterwards.

Each of you in turn share your experience of your first period—what was happening at that time, what you knew or didn't know about periods, what kind of acknowledgement you got, if any—while the others listen. What positive things would you have liked your parents or guardian to have said? Perhaps that you're special, beautiful, smart, funny, hard-working, creative, perfect just as you are, great at standing up to injustice, or a good friend. Imagine that you are that young girl. Your friends will now speak those positive things to you, adding their own affirmations of you as well. Perhaps they can give you a flower as a symbolic gift as they speak. Just drink it all in and say thanks at the end. And when you're ready move on to the next person.

Allow at least 30 minutes for each of you to go through the whole process—approximately twenty minutes for the sharing and ten minutes for hearing the positive statements. And have a box of tissues on hand as this exercise can be quite moving.

If none of your friends want to do the ritual you can do it on your own. Prepare the space in the same way, light the candle and with the photo in front of you write in your journal what it was like and what you would have preferred. Then speak out loud to that photo and tell her (you!) all the positive things you needed to hear about yourself and didn't.

One woman who had grown up in a very chaotic family instinctively felt that she needed to have a menarche ceremony to help her heal. She created it with the assistance of the psychotherapist she was seeing at the time.

Menarche for Maree was a non-event. Her mum treated it so matter of factly that Maree didn't get the kind of intimate, tender care she needed in that moment. Subsequently, menstruation never felt special to her either—it was something that you just put up with as you continued on with business as usual. After doing the menarche ceremony all that changed. It was as though she had connected into a deeper place in herself and menstruation now feels special and magical.

While depression can have multiple causes, making sure a girl has a positive experience at her first period can be a vital step in ensuring she grows up feeling good about herself and her life.

Slow is the new black

One of the reasons that periods can seem like a hassle is because they can slow you down. You may feel more tired, and want to slow down or do less. This is a healthy reminder from your body of the importance of having slow time to stay healthy and connected to yourself.

Zipping through your days at speed can be quite a high. But when you continually move faster than is comfortable for your body and your psyche's capacity to digest experience, stress builds. You can end up feeling weird, scrambled, maybe a bit shut down and deadened or emotionally all over the place, and you lose the capacity to respond in healthy ways. It's like jetlag of the soul. At speed all you can do is react rather than respond, which isn't constructive or healthy for you or anyone else.

The Slow Movement, which began in Italy, celebrates the pleasures of going slow, of taking time. From its origins in relation to food and cooking, the movement now embraces slow cities, slow education, slow sex, slow money and slow exercise. It values cyclical life and a leisurely pace, emphasising the importance of allowing each thing to unfold and flourish in its own right time.

Being slow means that you control the rhythms of your own life.
CARLO PETRINI, SLOW MOVEMENT FOUNDER

Have you felt the pull inward as winter approaches and wanted to stay in, knit, read and watch TV? And when spring comes suddenly felt the urge to get out there, start a new exercise program, clear the junk out of your cupboards and create space? Or maybe noticed how sometimes that it's just not the right timing to move on something and yet at other times nothing will stop you from going for it? That's you being in touch with your sense of 'timing'. Everything in cyclical life has its own timing. In farming 'slow' is about letting chickens roam and scratch in the sun as they grow naturally rather than being force-fed growth hormones to speed up the process.

The Slow Movement is about *improving* the quality of your life. As Carlo Petrini, one of its founders, said: 'Being slow means that you control the rhythms of your own life. You decide how fast you have to go in any given context . . . what we are fighting for is the right to determine your own tempo.'[5]

Today, the clock governs nearly everything we do but this doesn't always fit with the cyclical timing of nature and your body. Generally speaking, your body's pace will always feel slower. To the relentlessly doing speed-lover in you, slow will always feel too slow; but slowing down can open you up to a whole new experience of life, one that gets lost at speed. When you don't slow down some of the time it may be forced on you. You may get sick and have to take time off work, make costly mistakes because you're overtired, or end up feeling depressed and this zaps your will to do anything.

Sometimes to be faster, you have to be slower.[6]
JACKIE STEWART, FORMULA ONE DRIVER

Janey was flying high running her own business as well as buying a home, followed in quick succession by the purchase of a second property

> Caring for your menstrual cycle is a hidden key to creating a more ordered, connected, productive and meaningful life—for really being in the hum and flow of things.

as an investment. It was the classic 'having it all' scenario until her health collapsed. A driven person, she had forgotten to factor in the needs of her body and spirit and eventually they spoke in no uncertain terms. She was unable to work for two years and consequently lost her business and investments.

Allowing for more spaciousness and time in your life to follow your own rhythm does wonders for all aspects of you. If keeping yourself busy is your usual mode of operating, slowing down may feel a bit weird and even boring. That's quite a normal reaction to have initially when you're changing gear. Just go gently with yourself, trust in the new pace and gradually you'll feel more aware, alive, sensitive and responsive and maybe even zinging with creative ideas—these are the signs of being connected.

Following natural rhythms may feel like a luxury you can't afford

In most technically advanced countries the world is starting to look a lot more woman friendly. Women have far more opportunity and freedom to achieve success economically, culturally and politically. The changing nature of work means that women's talents can flourish even more. Nonetheless, professional life and the double shift at home place high demands on women.

Given the pressures of modern life, following your natural rhythms may feel like a luxury you can't afford. Dealing with the conflicting demands of life can be challenging. In such a climate, the Pill may look attractive, especially if you suffer from menstrual problems. However, the solution to shut down or artificially regulate your cycle could prove in the long term much more expensive and time consuming, rather like the high cost of dealing with the fallout from agribusiness farming, which runs into the billions each year.

Creating coherence

Coherence is a state in which all the separate parts of you fit together to form a harmonious whole, and that coherence creates a far more dynamic and powerful you. It's a bit like saying the whole is greater than the sum of its parts. A coherent system is an energy efficient system. You need less energy to achieve much greater results than you would if you're scattered and uncentred.

Taking the Pill so you can feel freer is contradictory. A feeling of freedom naturally arises when you're comfortable with yourself and connected to your body. This is coherence. Katie's really enjoying being in touch with her cycle after years on the Pill. 'Awareness of the cycle is a resource,' she said, 'like having a direct line to what's happening inside myself and gives me choice. I can play to that observation and be more responsive . . . it's loosened up something in me. I'm more sympathetic to the mood I'm in at work and cooperate with that. I'm more thoughtful about what I now undertake. It's such a relief . . . I'm really loving it. I never used to understand in all those self-help books what they meant by empowerment, I was a bit cynical, but now I just get it!'

The challenge is to value your own timing. Ironically, the menstrual cycle, rather than being the enemy, graces you with marvellous assets that help you to know your own timing. It keeps you grounded in your body, and therefore more connected with your true self—the very thing you need for dealing with a high pressured, ambitious life. Caring for your menstrual cycle is a hidden key to creating a more ordered, connected, productive and meaningful life—for really being in the hum and flow of things.

Menstruation can still be a bit painful now I'm off the Pill, but I quite like that, it makes me feel connected to my body and myself. Menstruation opens up in me that raw female goddess energy, it's indescribable—a loving, nurturing, powerful energy, that reminds me that I have the ability to create life—which means I can do anything.

REBECCA, 24

CHAPTER 22

YOUR VERY OWN FEED-BACK LOOP

Your body is a field of living information, with feedback loops constantly in place.[1]
DEEPAK CHOPRA

Cassie, 24, suffered from period pain until she realised how much her lifestyle impacted her body. By managing her workload better, eating well and slowing down when she has her period, she now has less pain. Recently she took an extended holiday and by the end of her trip she had no period pain at all. Back home this continued for a month or two before the stress of a new job and moving house saw the pain creep back. Now she really gets how stress can affect her wellbeing, and how her cycle can alert her to that. 'Wow, it's such a blessing. I'm really proud of my body that it gives me feedback,' she exclaimed. Your menstrual cycle is an ever-changing, finely tuned system. Responding to your inner and outer environment, it gives you monthly feedback on how you're managing life physically and emotionally.

A Traditional Chinese Medicine practitioner can use all the signs and symptoms of your menstrual cycle—whether it's a short or long cycle, heavy or scant bleeding, or the quality of the blood—as a diagnostic tool. As a psychotherapist I find that by knowing about a woman's experience of her cycle, I can get indications about that woman's strengths, challenges and vulnerabilities, that might also include her ability to assert herself, self-esteem levels and how well she's handling relationships.

Premenstrual syndrome can indicate that you're a bit rundown, your diet's poor, that you need to assert yourself more or that you're not really going for what you want in life. Periods will stop when the body is very stressed or not sufficiently nourished, such as when a woman suffers from an eating disorder or overexercises. Women with chronic health conditions may find that they flair up just before bleeding, and if you're excessively rundown you could be more prone to getting colds or flu at that time too. This is your wonderful body giving you feedback through the cycle.

When I began reading Christiane Northrup's Women's Bodies, Women's Wisdom, *I fell in love with the amazing feminine cycle. I was on the Pill for seven years, which acted as a wonderful suppressant—suppressing my emotions, intuition and most importantly my LIBIDO. I'm still recovering all of these things five years after stopping the Pill.*

TARYN, 29

Turning the spotlight on yourself

Have you noticed how at ovulation you can be more focused on the outer world—your work, family and friends? As you draw into your period that focus shifts. It's as though the spotlight comes off others for a while and onto you. At your period you tune more deeply into your inner self, and the outer stuff can almost feel like an irritant or a burden. Your body, through the cycle, is reminding you to take time for yourself.

In the premenstrual phase—that's approximately a week or so before bleeding—the immune system appears to be slightly more vulnerable, your senses and feelings more heightened, your intuition stronger and you might have more vivid dreams. You can't repress stuff in the same way and you'll see and feel things you couldn't before. This is both powerful and healthy.

> Your menstrual cycle is an ever-changing, finely tuned system. Responding to your inner and outer environment, it gives you monthly feedback on how you're managing life physically and emotionally.

If you've been cranky with someone and you've held back from speaking, you may now find yourself expressing that frustration. If you're not happy with any part of your life you may feel overly critical of yourself or depressed. Take it as a sign that you need to re-examine your priorities.

Feeling overwhelmed can indicate that you've just got too much on or that you're overtired, not necessarily that you're en route to a psychological breakdown! It's also important to remember that some change of mood in that second half of the cycle is simply part of the process of changing from being very 'out there' to being more connected to yourself. It's normal to have these fluctuations and being more accepting of the ups and downs eases them.

Some women find old hurts surface before their period, making them feel more vulnerable. Perhaps you suffer from an overly critical boss or a friend who's let you down badly or, more distressingly, suffered from sexual or emotional abuse. Your feelings of hurt can manifest themselves in being easily upset, not feeling good about yourself, depression, addictive behaviour, anger or criticism of yourself or others. You may find professional counselling support can help deal with these issues, particularly healing past abuse.

If you've changed the areas in your life that were stressing you out, then there is far less to rise to the surface premenstrually. That's what I'm finding anyway. I still have some PMS grouchiness, but not such huge traumas.

FRAN, 32

It's time to get real

Crankiness and feelings of anger can be great motivators. Anger is a fabulous force *but* it can come out in somewhat wild and destructive ways. It's a power and, as with all powers, it can be used or abused. Your challenge is to learn how to harness this force. You may need to apologise for how you spoke to your best friend or a colleague at work in a fit of anger. Once you've done that take a look at the essential truth behind your outburst. If you, or those around you, dismiss what you say as 'just premenstrual', something important in you is also being dismissed.

If you tend to be more strongly assertive, angry or critical, consider that you're a frustrated leader or change agent and that you're just not utilising that energy. You could be in a job that doesn't utilise all your talents, or value what you have to offer. Or you're repressing your opinions or ideas and need to step forward more with them. When you don't attend to these things, your power will fester inside, only to turn up again next month with more reactivity. Not a good look!

If this sounds like you, then it's time to take yourself in hand. Make a list of everything you'd love to be doing. It doesn't matter how wild and impossible your ideas are, love them all. If there are themes emerging, chunk them into categories—relationships, work, family, living arrangements, your 'big secret dream' ideas. What are your priorities? Start with what you feel is the most important. Find small things you can do every day that lead towards that goal. It might be a phone call, a browse on the net, or brainstorming with a friend. Keep going with the small steps.

You'll feel like you're doing something towards achieving your goals, which creates a good feeling and further motivation to keep going. And as you take one step, usually another reveals itself in a way that wouldn't have happened if you hadn't made the first move.

Once you make a commitment to change, however modestly, a strange magic occurs—experiencing things like synchronicities and chance meetings—that open the way. This happened to Fran. She felt like she was becoming a monster each month just before her period. And she was particularly distressed at how she could turn her frustrations on her husband. Not happy with her job or the long commuting hours, she decided she had to leave. Giving herself permission to not work for a short period, she was determined in that time to find work that felt meaningful and aligned with her own values, even turning down a couple of offers for well paid work in the same field she had just left. While out walking one day with her husband a beautiful old building caught their attention. Fran was curious to know more. That curiosity led to being employed by the company that works from that building. She loves her work now. It's creative and at times demanding but, because she feels respected and stimulated, she's rising to meet the challenges. Her main difficulty when she has her period now is tiredness, which alerts her to balance her own needs with those of the job.

If you find it hard to make changes by yourself, why not consider hiring a life coach or team up with a buddy?

There's a saying that the people who are successful are the ones who have hung in after everyone else has given up. Instead of cursing your PMS, you'll be using it as a catalyst for changing the aspects of your life that aren't working—for getting real.

It's not all personal

Our bodies aren't just giving us feedback about ourselves but are also responding to the world around us—the levels of noise, the pace of modern life, the amount of technology, as well as the emotional impact of global violence and environmental upheaval. All these influences are wearing, and at times overwhelming, for our bodies and spirits.

To protect ourselves we often numb out a bit, becoming insensitive and developing compassion fatigue. As you come into the premenstrual or 'getting real' phase of the cycle—the time when you are more sensitive—the parts of you that may be numb or shut down start to wake up. You're coming to your senses. It's a bit like the feeling of the anaesthetic wearing off after you've had your tooth numbed for dental work—your tooth feels tender and sore as it comes back to life. In the same way you can feel a bit tender and vulnerable in those days before bleeding. This is actually a healthy sign of your emotional aliveness. Certain things may indeed seem intolerable, and rightly so. Instead of seeing PMS as a personal problem or medicating it, use the drive constructively to change things.

Amy, who is outspoken and passionate, found herself unable to keep quiet at a new job. As a freelance make-up artist in the music and film industry, she took a temporary position in a photographic studio. The photographer made sleazy remarks while photographing a young pregnant woman. Amy couldn't take it and complained to management. It was a risk and there was no guarantee they'd listen, but it was the day before her period and she wasn't going to be silenced. Management did listen. They wanted to employ women like Amy who cared about these issues, and their other studios were alerted to the problem. Her stance would benefit every woman coming in to be photographed and the business as a whole.

You might find yourself doing the opposite, becoming easily overwhelmed and needing to 'disappear' from the world a little rather than confront it. While you might feel like you're not making any contribution at work or at home, don't push yourself to be something you're not. Withdrawing, resting, enjoying some silence and restoring your spirit are equally important things. When you model this, it helps others to value time out too. In this quiet time you'll be able to tap in to your intuition and sense new possibilities that were unavailable to you while 'out there'. Rosie, a highly sensitive and creative woman, has to avoid watching the news around her period as well as being less social. Everything just feels too much for her: 'It's like I'm feeling for the world at that time,' she reflects.

The canary in the mineshaft

How you're faring with your periods may also be giving you feedback about the unsafe levels of environmental pollutants around you. Like miners in the early days who used canaries to alert them to any changes in air quality—the birds started to keel over if the air was toxic—your heavy bleeding, endometriosis, period pain, PMS, fibroids or polycystic ovarian syndrome are, in part, an indication of the high levels of environmental toxicity that you're subjected to.

Tens of thousands of chemicals have been created since World War II and every year approximately 2000 new compounds are released, very few of which are systematically screened.[2] Many of these can disrupt the endocrine system and the menstrual cycle. A number of the chemicals in pesticides and plastics act as 'oestrogen mimics'. They can attach themselves to oestrogen receptors in our bodies and upset our natural hormonal balance. Along with these and other toxic chemicals, electromagnetic radiation emanating from all our technology is also impacting on our health.

As menstruating women we get monthly 'canary in the mineshaft' feedback about how we're handling the environmental load and a strong signal to remove toxic substances from our environment for the sake of both our health and that of others.

When 'No' means 'Yes'

A vital part of taking care of yourself both physically and emotionally involves being able to comfortably assert yourself—asking for what you want and saying no to those things that don't support you, whether it's the behaviour of a friend, a job you don't like or products that are environmentally unsound.

In the days leading up to your period, your patience levels may drop precipitously. This doesn't mean that you've suddenly morphed into a horrible, selfish person. It's merely a signal that you need to keep your energy more for you now. And this will involve you saying 'No' to others and 'Yes' to yourself more often.

> Women need to understand that it is OK to be vulnerable at certain times without letting it overwhelm them. It's OK to say no—for many women, this is the most difficult technique to master of all.[3]
> JANE USSHER, PROFESSOR OF WOMEN'S HEALTH PSYCHOLOGY

If you're not comfortable with saying what you can and can't do, or asking for what you need, then you may come unstuck and experience some of the classic PMS symptoms of irritability and feeling over-whelmed. Conversely, as you learn to feel OK about your wants and needs and can stand up for them, you'll feel less reactive. And the more you can assert yourself, the stronger your personal boundaries and sense of self will be and the less emotional reactivity you'll have. The premenstrual phase can help you to stand up for your own needs and take better care of yourself. It affects everything in your life—improving your relationships, making you more effective in your job and clearer and more determined about achieving your life goals. Constantly being a 'yes' person to everyone else's demands won't serve this purpose—you need to develop the ability to say no to others and yes to yourself.

Are you really nourishing yourself?

If you're not up for all that inner reflection and challenging the world, the good news is that making sure you have a great diet can have an amazing effect on your menstrual problems. Our bodies can be remarkably long suffering but will eventually present their bill if they don't get sufficient care and nourishment. Generally speaking menstruation is a regular moment of truth. Eating a poor diet, drinking excessive alcohol—or any at all if you're highly sensitive—taking drugs, doing little exercise, not getting enough sleep will all stress your body. You can easily end up feeling emotionally jangled premenstrually, as well as at other times.

When Cassie, in her early twenties, stopped menstruating she was worried. It turned out Cassie was stressed to the eyeballs. 'There was no balance in my life. I was studying and working very hard, moods all over the place, it was totally extreme. And it was a hard spot to get out of,' she confessed. Her body was giving her very clear feedback that her lifestyle wasn't working. Fortunately she listened to her body, taking care to restore balance through proper nourishing care. 'There wasn't enough soul-food type stuff in my life,' Cassie admits. 'I realised that I needed balance in every aspect to get hormonal balance. I started doing more yoga and less weight and cardio training. I started eating meat and introducing good fats, as I was well aware that my hormones are made up of fat and protein and I wasn't eating enough of these. I started socialising more with friends instead of studying and ignoring my need for "fun". I was too hard on my body and it was crying out for a little nourishment.' Now Cassie menstruates regularly and gives herself time off when she bleeds. She sees this as her precious rebalancing time.

Eight ways to ease difficult periods

1. Eat regular nourishing meals so your blood sugar levels don't plummet.
2. Cut out sugar and white flour products and reduce your coffee, tea and alcohol intake because they can make you reactive and tetchy.
3. Get sufficient exercise and rest.
4. Respect the feelings that do emerge as meaningful even if you don't always fully understand them.
5. Keep a journal in which you write, dream, mull, draw and doodle when you're troubled, want to work things out, figure out your needs *and* celebrate your successes.
6. Practise asserting yourself on smaller issues the whole month long, so that you feel there's balance in your relationships.
7. Pause, think and feel before responding to a request.
8. Do something special for yourself when you bleed.

The 'no feedback' system

I was diagnosed with endometriosis at age 25 and cervical dysplasia [abnormal cells on the surface of the cervix] at age 33. I believe such reproductive problems have been influenced by the Pill's use. The suppression of my natural cycle (and subsequent inability to track or detect underlying conditions) kept me in a state of 'fertility limbo' and it wasn't until I stopped using the Pill that I became aware that my reproductive system needed urgent attention.

LILLIAN, 36

When you're on the Pill you don't have the benefit of this feedback as it shuts down your natural hormonal system, and lays the ground for further hormonal upheavals and general health problems as you've heard about in earlier chapters.

You may be taking the Pill, or be drawn to take it, because you have *too much* feedback going on, and neither you nor your doctor knows any other way to treat your menstrual problems. The Pill may give you crucial relief. If you're on the Pill because of menstrual problems, or are considering it for this purpose, begin to look at alternatives such as dietary changes. Eat lots of fresh vegetables and fruit and avoid soft drinks and refined products. Reduce environmental pollutants by using only body products with natural ingredients. Practise stress management techniques like yoga, meditation and charting your menstrual cycle, so that you can begin to value and flow with the different seasons of your body.

Ultimately, whether it's the state of your overall health, how you're travelling emotionally, or the stresses of your daily life, your marvellous endocrine system is reporting back to you monthly. If you take the Pill you shut down this inner compass and create further health challenges for yourself.

CHAPTER 23

TAPPING YOUR INTUITION

You have a deep inner knowing in yourself that can guide you to what's right and not right for you. When you're in touch with this inner wisdom your life can feel more meaningful and your direction clearer. The more you listen to your feelings, even when you don't fully understand them, and trust your gut instincts, the stronger your intuition, your inner knowing, will be. Your menstrual cycle is a wonderful way for you to develop the intuitive you.

In Native American tradition there's a beautiful saying that at her first period a girl meets her wisdom. Through her menstruating years she practises her wisdom, and at menopause she becomes her wisdom. We 'practise our wisdom' by paying attention to the feedback we get during our period. It helps us value our feelings, instincts and intuitions, giving us a more expanded intelligence alongside our intellectual self.

I feel incredibly sexual, powerful, energetic and driven in the first half of my cycle, till around day sixteen. Day 22 onwards I feel more of a lull and a slight 'down-ness'. Sometimes this can be reflected emotionally with sadness, sometimes I just feel calm and grounded—like a profound 'knowingness' about myself.

MICHELLE, 35

Being in touch with yourself

The simple act of charting your cycle in the way we've described in Chapter 20 is the first step towards tapping your intuitive self. Like focusing on your breath if you meditate, knowing where you are in your cycle helps you feel more grounded and comfortable in your own skin. As you do this, you'll also learn to recognise when you're ovulating and when your period is due. Knowing what your body is doing can feel just plain good and quite empowering. The process of charting your cycle is like keeping a journal, a time-honoured tradition for being in touch with yourself, in which you record all the deeper stuff going on in your life, the highs and the lows, the challenges and the wins. By combining journal writing with charting your cycle, you'll have an even more potent tool.

The simple act of writing a few words a day allowed Clare to begin to take herself seriously. It was as though the different feelings and thoughts 'spoke' to her, indicating her various needs and goals. They became signposts to what was most important.

Your sensations and emotions are a form of intelligence that speak to you about your true path. Sometimes they can speak an uncomfortable, rocking-the-boat sort of truth. Or they can seem irrational or silly to our 'rational' minds. You could be in denial about some aspect of your life and in the 'getting real' phase find yourself bursting into tears or being overly reactive 'for no reason', therefore dismissing the feelings as 'just premenstrual'.

Your feelings are giving you guidance. Even if it feels scary to act, at least start to acknowledge to yourself the truth of what you're feeling. When you dismiss or trivialise your feelings, you often end up overriding your instincts, hunches and intuitions, and lose connection to your wise inner voice.

Off the Pill I feel much more alive, much more in tune with my body and my senses. I feel that my intuition is developing and that I am in a much better position to make decisions about my health.

ELLEN, 26

Learning to trust your feelings and using them as guidance for your life takes time. It's an art, which means it's an imperfect business—you may get it wrong sometimes. Wishful thinking can be confused with true feelings. Getting overly emotional can distort your inner compass. However, with time, awareness and respect you'll notice a greater confidence in your inner sensing and knowing.

You may be doing your best to *avoid* feeling what's happening on the inside and the Pill would be great, thank you very much! This is understandable, but avoiding your feelings doesn't work long term. Feelings don't vanish. They get repressed until they reappear in a more extreme shape or form as depression, illness, anger or addiction. Getting counselling support can help you to gently and slowly like yourself more. As you do that you'll be able to access your feelings with greater ease.

Listening to your dreams

Your dreams are a marvellous doorway into your inner self and the more you are in touch with them the more you build your inner wisdom. You may like to chart your dreams throughout the cycle. Particular types of dreams or dream characters often turn up at particular phases of the cycle. Without fail Ali would be confronted each month before her period by dreams of thugs and mafia-type figures threatening her life. Over time the dreams shifted so that she was fighting back more and even threatening them. In real life she was learning about how to channel her power, not to become a literal thug of course, but learning to be more direct and fearless in expressing herself.

Working with dream images can give you real insight as they did for Ali. And the dreams around your period can have more 'standout' significance. Sometimes they are very moving, giving you penetrating insight, or they can even be quite prescient, indicating something about your future. You might also dream of blood or something red just before your period—a useful reminder it's due. Adding dream work to your techniques can provide another layer to charting your cycle, one that will allow you to learn more juicy stuff about the wealth of your inner resources.

Lisa, who we met earlier, loved recording her dreams and had a morning ritual of writing in her journal upon waking. But one morning, after having started the Pill again, she found herself lying there with pen in hand drawing a complete blank. Her dreams had become such a rich and vital tool in her quest for self-discovery and personal growth, this 'side-effect' of zero dream recall was intolerable. It became another reason for her to stop the Pill.

Exploring your dreams

To work and play with your dreams it helps to write them down, otherwise they can be forgotten very quickly. Don't worry if you can't recall the whole dream, because even a fragment of memory can be useful. Often the simple act of recording it in words or drawings can give you that 'click' of intuitive understanding about what your dream is revealing to you.

Sally Gillespie, author of *Living the Dream*, suggests asking yourself the following questions to help you unfold your dream messages:

1. What was on your mind the day before your dream?
2. What were you doing in the dream?
3. What were you feeling in your dream?
4. Who or what did you encounter in your dream?
5. What was the strongest part of the dream?
6. How did you feel when you woke up?

Writing down the answers to these questions after recording your dream will help you move more into your dream landscape, as well as relate what you see there to your current external life.[1]

Your 'tent' time

In the red tent, the truth is known.[2]

ANITA DIAMANT, AUTHOR

Another way to access your intuition is to take 'tent' time. Traditionally women in many cultures would separate themselves from their communities when they menstruated. They would retreat to a special hut, tent or place in nature where they could relinquish the demands of everyday life to nourish their spiritual life and vision for their community. 'Tent' time is a way of talking about the space of menstruation, the time for resting and listening to your inner wisdom.

Emma, speaking at a businesswomen's forum, encouraged the participants to use their cycle for creating success. 'I taught them how to plan their work schedule around their cycle for ultimate productivity . . . to book up their schedules at ovulation, get out and network and close their sales. On the opposite end of the scale, their tent time (they loved that) was reserved for the gentle/non-client contact jobs. They were elated that someone gave them permission to take some chill-out time at their period and go off into their tent for a few days.' Not only would they get well-deserved rest they'd also open the door wider to their intuition.

You can claim *your* 'tent' time by taking some personal space for yourself. If you can really let go when the blood starts to flow, you can experience a delicious feeling of connectedness. It is as though you've been restored to the core of your being and have access to a deeper source of knowledge. Ideas and solutions to difficult problems can literally flood in or well up out of nowhere. Simply drink it in.

When a friend rang Debbie to ask what she was doing she said, 'Lying on my couch.' Her friend assumed that she was bored with nothing to do. Debbie insisted that she was doing something very lovely 'lying on her couch'. As she was having her period she was really enjoying just blissing out on 'me time'.

I felt really wise all day (the first day of the bleed). I could engage with anyone's problems. I was in this place where I could dish out pearls of wisdom. I was doing what I was supposed to be doing. I felt very present, standing in power and love.

AMY, 37

Your inner psychic

While you might like to go to a psychic occasionally, to get some direction about your life, did you know that when you bleed you can access your own psychic ability more easily? Some women who are already highly sensitive can experience quite strong psychic phenomena around their periods. Women who have this capacity but are not aware of it may feel over-whelmed or quite despairing just before bleeding. Without knowing it their premenstrual moodiness may be their visionary capacity kicking in.

Jessie has what she can only describe as 360-degree vision just before her period. 'It's like I'm outside my mind and can see everything around me. It's almost too much, I don't know how to block it out. I can see into what's happening for people. I used to think that something was wrong with me that this happened.' Because no-one understood and supported her sensitivity Jessie used alcohol and later antidepressants to manage that time, until she understood what was going on. Now she's coming off the antidepressants and is slowly learning how to make this heightened sensitivity work for her.

Julia, a naturopathic student, found herself in the same boat, until she realised what was going on. 'It all makes sense,' Julia said. 'I'm clair-voyant, and each month before my period everything feels terrible.' Julia would end up an emotional mess and ring her mother in despair. Her mother eventually realised that this happened just before Julia bled. For women like Julia, this understanding alone can make an enormous difference to their sense of self and their wellbeing.

If you're such a woman, don't push or overexpose yourself in the days just before your period. Eat well, avoid stimulants such as sugar, coffee and alcohol, and get plenty of rest. Instead of feeling despair or bleakness you'll gradually feel more grounded and empowered in your psychic and intuitive ability, and be able to use it constructively. Your friends will be coming to you instead when you bleed for their psychic reading.

Whether this is you or not, you might like to protect yourself during this highly sensitive and charged time of the month, so imagine you have an invisible 'tent' or some other secret buffer around you that gives you a sense of being safe. You might find yourself holding back and watching more, keeping your own counsel, feeling a delicious inner privacy. This can be surprisingly restful, creating an inner softness and calmness that will have you knowing just what to say and do.

Tune out to tune in

To get the full benefit of inspiration and vision, take time out from everything, including technology. Switch off your mobile, computer and TV. You'll live without them, we promise you! Start off by chilling out over a cup of tea, walking in nature, shutting your bedroom door and curling up under the doona or soaking in a bath. The point is to drop all your usual agendas and 'to do' lists and relax. As you tune out the usual distractions and noise, you'll find you naturally tune in to your inspired self—to your inner guidance. If you're used to a lot of activity and need this to feel OK, then it can initially seem a bit weird or boring. Do it anyway, and hang in there. The more you do it the more the mysterious magic of menstruation can steal over you. It might be a warm inner feeling of OK-ness or simple relief.

In Native American tradition there's a beautiful saying that at her first period a girl meets her wisdom. Through her menstruating years she practises her wisdom, and at menopause she becomes her wisdom.

There's a practice in the Native American tradition called the vision quest, in which you go into nature on your own and fast for a number of days to gain visions and spiritual guidance for your life. It's practised by men and is also used as an initiation rite for boys becoming men. Today, in the West, many men and women have adopted this practice. While it's a wonderful thing to do, what is rarely understood is that women don't need to go bush and fast, they simply have to withdraw and be quiet and still when they bleed—menstruation is a woman's way of vision-questing. And the more silence and emptiness you give yourself, the more profound the experience will be.

Visions come in different ways at menstruation. You could get a clear picture in your mind of what you need to be doing, or a powerful dream that leaves a special feeling inside you, helping you to be more accepting of who you are or what's happening in your life. Or you could simply have a sure knowingness that a certain action must be taken. Suddenly you are clear about what must be done.

I hated taking the Pill. It felt like I came out of a daze when I finally got off it after five years on . . . and would never ever use it again. It felt like it took my deepest parts away.

MELI, 34

'Bleeding' on it

Just as you might say to someone 'I'll sleep on that and get back to you', you can also 'bleed on' a problem to get a resolution. Menstruation is the classic time for figuring things out, although you don't so much 'think' through the problem as listen for the answer arising in you.

Anna had hit crunch time with her PhD. She'd already done a fair amount of work on it but there was still a long way to go and she was seriously thinking of quitting. She was getting married and had sudden doubts about that too. Two huge decisions to make, she chose to use the 'bleed on it' method to find what was really right for her. Giving herself a couple of menstrual months, she felt all the conflicting tensions without trying to resolve them. As she bled she would let go and feel the deep knowing of her being rise in her. It was an undeniable yes to both. And getting in touch with that deeper sureness helped her face the challenges involved with greater confidence.

Here's how it works: hold any dilemma or question inside you keeping open to any thoughts or feelings that you have about it and, as you come into menstruation, let go of all effort to solve it, almost forgetting about the issue. Feel your whole being relax and surrender; rest, sleep, blob out and gradually, as the bleeding eases, you'll find yourself in a place of greater clarity. The answer you're seeking is suddenly very obvious or you may simply feel a quiet, sure recognition of what's right. If you rush out into the world too quickly and lose this intimacy with yourself, you may miss the moment.

You need two types of attention now. Your normal, everyday attention focusing on the business of the world and a second attention that's operating on a deeper register, so to speak, quietly feeling and observing subtle details. We do this rather well generally, it's part of our multi-tasking capacity. It's like using your peripheral vision. Your second attention will allow you to catch the direction or instructions from your inner being.

Loving yourself

As I work with the cycle I feel more and more loving and accepting of myself.
I feel close to truth.

CLARE, 22

We can all struggle with loving ourselves at times. If I was thinner, smarter, had bigger or smaller boobs, had more of this or less of that, I'd finally be OK. Accepting ourselves in spite of the bits that we struggle with is, of course, what we need to do most of all.

The simple act of valuing your cycle is a wonderful way to help you accept yourself as a woman. Isabelle, a child protection specialist, found that once she started to use the cycle as her means for inner guidance she felt much better about herself and more connected to other women. As she said, 'I feel empowered by the cycle now and have a deeper understanding of who I am and what it is to be a woman.' When she bleeds she feels more grounded and aware, allowing herself to be more present and therefore more skilful in her challenging and highly sensitive role interviewing girls and young women who have been abused.

The greater your capacity for liking yourself, caring for your health and valuing your cyclical nature, the stronger that kind, inner, wise voice can become, directing you to what is right for you. Through the monthly pattern of the cycle your wisdom grows and transforms like the caterpillar becoming a butterfly. When a caterpillar wraps itself in a chrysalis en route to becoming a butterfly, first it dissolves, becoming mush. Within this new cells emerge and, through the interconnections they make with each other, develop into a butterfly. Think of the butterfly as being your inner wisdom. Each month as you come into menstruation and feel yourself wanting to withdraw, your mind becoming dreamy, it's like the caterpillar going into its chrysalis. When you let go it's your version of dissolving into mush and out of this your 'butterfly' of new inspirations and deepening awareness can emerge.

Perhaps it's time for you to see your period as a sacred or special time, whatever that might mean for you. When you do, out of nowhere you'll start to feel easier with yourself and surer about who you are and what it is that you need to do. This is your wisdom growing in you and you growing into your wisdom.

CHAPTER 24

DISCOVERING NATURAL CALM

The feeling that came over me was glorious, like nectar in the veins. It was like the feeling you get after really great sex. It was wonderful. That evening the blood started to flow.

MAREE, 45

The secret that some women have already stumbled on and relish every month is that menstruation can be a place of soothing, stilling, even bliss. With some care and attention it can become your natural, inbuilt de-stressing zone.

Maree discovered this after doing Alexandra's workshop. It was a day that she didn't have to take the children to school. She could feel her period was about to begin. Normally she'd just have gone straight ahead with her usual schedule, but since she'd just done the workshop on menstruation, she thought she'd try out Alexandra's suggestions. 'I cancelled everything,' she said, 'and sat wrapped in my doona looking out at the garden. The feeling that came over me was glorious, like nectar in the veins. It was like the feeling you get after really great sex. It was wonderful. That evening the blood started to flow.'

In our 24/7 lifestyle it's more important than ever to create islands of calm—timeout in which to release tension and simply 'be' for a while. Just as you can't go without sleep for too long, so your psyche can't go for too long without some quality downtime. In the menstrual cycle, your period is the classic cyclic 'downtime'. In fact, if menstruation were a product you could purchase it would be called Natural Calm, and make billions!

The sad thing is that when you're on the Pill, you lose this special moment as the breakthrough bleed on the Pill is not a normal menstruation. It is as it sounds, merely a breakthrough bleed, so it doesn't have the same delicious impact a true period can bring you. We can't help but wonder, apart from other health issues, what the longer-term emotional effects are for women on the Pill who are deprived of their natural release and calm.

I try to take a 'sick' day if my cycle feels very tiring and honour the mysterious energetic process that happens by doing little and just being.

KELLY, 30

Creating calm for optimum brain performance

Science seems to agree about our need for more quiet time. Recently neurobiologist Leo Chalupa proposed a national day of absolute solitude—no verbal exchange with anyone—as the best antidote for our overtaxed, overstuffed brains, and the ideal way to attain optimal brain performance.[1]

Researcher and psychologist Peter Suedfeld came to similar conclusions, stating that everyone was chronically stimulated, socially and physically, and that we 'are probably operating at a stimulation level higher than that for which our species evolved'. His remedy? More time alone. Two other scientists also found that attentive listening to silence helps one's brain to focus.[2] You can also effectively add conscious menstruation to that list of ways to attain 'optimal brain performance'.

Billi notices that the feeling of calm can steal over her about two days before she bleeds. Any angst she's been having about things in her life seems to slip away, and along with the calm comes a feeling of oneness and love—like the feeling of being 'in love'. And then as her blood starts to flow, she has the sensation of release and letting go. She feels herself unloading gently, allowing her to refocus for the next month.

The Sabbath of women
In her book *Honouring Menstruation: A Time of Self Renewal*, Lara Owen called menstruation the Sabbath of women. In Babylonian times there was a festival called Sabat to celebrate the goddess of the moon, Ishtar. It occurred at full moon, when it was said the goddess menstruated. Work, travel and eating cooked food were prohibited for women and men on this day. Those distant days of rest linked to the moon and menstruation were the origins of the Christian Sunday and the Jewish Sabbath.[3]

The calm, love and trust hormone

There are chemical changes that happen in your body that may be linked to these feelings of calm. Oxytocin has been called the love hormone because it engenders feelings of love, calm and belonging. It's released during sexual activity, male and female orgasm, birth and breastfeeding, as well as when we're touching, hugging, and sharing a meal.[4] Orgasm causes oxytocin levels to rise from three to five times higher than normal, creating that delicious glow of closeness and tenderness that is experienced after lovemaking. And just as contractions of the uterus release oxytocin during lovemaking, birthing and breastfeeding, so it is released at menstruation, when the uterus also contracts.

It's always such a blessed relief when I get my period, like a dear and familiar friend who visits me. I really find it quite comforting. I feel soft and tender.
SHUSHANN, 47

Natalie Angier in her book *Woman: An Intimate Geography* describes a special moment on the day her period arrived: 'I was sitting in my living room, studying, and I felt an unaccountable surge of joy. I looked up from my book and was dazzled by the air. It was so clear, so purely transparent, that the objects in the room were sharply etched and proud against it, and yet it was as though I could see the air for the first time. It had become visible to me, molecule for molecule. My mind was focussed and free of anxiety. I felt for a moment as though I had taken the perfect drug, the one that has yet to be invented; call it Liberitium or Creativil.'[5]

This drug doesn't need to be invented. Our bodies create it at menstruation and at those other special times. It's possible for you to enjoy the benefits of this hormone when you give time and space to yourself when you bleed.

If you suffer from bad period pain you may find it hard to even imagine, let alone access, feelings of calm and bliss at this time. However, if you follow the tips at the end of the chapter and also put in place the self-care practices described in Chapters 27 and 28, you may start to experience less pain, and begin to experience inklings of the calm.

If you don't suffer overly at menstruation, you'll probably have experienced some relief and release when you bleed, but may not have experienced the kind of blissful feelings that we've described. You might also experience a wave of tiredness or just not wanting to do anything at all. Regard those feelings as the first tendrils of the calm and bliss wanting to embrace you, and with a little more space and quiet, this may start to flow more freely. However, if you try to keep going with your regular schedule while bleeding, you may just miss this lovely opportunity.

When you ignore your need to chill out or withdraw at this time, you may end up with classic PMS symptoms such as disorientation, dreaminess, fogginess, feeling overwhelmed and irritable as well as headaches and period pain. But if you can begin to see your period as a time to really change gear and take a break, the calm will find you.

Cassie, who we met earlier, is highly motivated and ambitious. As she likes to run every day and keeps herself very busy, she feels guilty if she isn't doing stuff. When she bled and felt the pull from inside to be quieter, she'd constantly push it aside. While it's great she's so motivated, ignoring her body's signal to slow down is not a smart idea. Since reading about the gifts of menstruation—how it keeps her in balance and in touch with herself—she has a completely new approach. 'Wow, I can have two days off when I bleed and not feel guilty. It's OK not to run on the day I bleed, and I have an excuse to go to bed at 9 pm. It helps me to care for my more vulnerable parts and it's nice to sit with that and dream.'

> Menstruation is profoundly grounding—that means feeling really connected to your whole self.

Why not slow down just before the period? Aim to make the first day of bleeding special. As for Cassie, that usually means allowing yourself some slack that day, such as not pushing yourself to do your usual exercise routine, dropping your to-do list, or trying to be there for your friends. It's a 'be kind to yourself' day—the day when you give ambition, drive and focus a rest, a day to receive rather than to give. Kathy came up with the acronym PLAY— Please Look After Yourself. So think of menstruation as PLAY time. It doesn't mean you can't do anything. You're no less functional or brilliant. It's simply that you deliver in a different way.

Amy came up with another marvellous idea, calling her period the time to 'raise the red flag'. She and her friends record in their mobiles approximately when their friends' periods are due. Their mobiles alert them to text or ring to see how their friend is doing, reminding them it's time to relax and checking whether they need any extra help, for example with children.

Menstruation is natural meditation

As menstruation draws you more surely into your body and feelings, it brings you into the present moment. Menstruation is profoundly grounding—that means feeling really connected to your whole self. The purpose of meditation is similar: to ground you in the present moment and in yourself. Menstruation offers that naturally when you're in tune with your body and not fighting against it. You're then able to do your work from a more centred place and this will allow you to experience that calm.

Even if you lead a very high-pressured life with barely a moment to yourself, with only a simple change in attitude, you'll start to get a taste of this. The next time you bleed take one minute before you plunge into your day and feel your body exactly as it is. Acknowledge quietly to yourself whatever it is you're noticing. Ask yourself: 'If I didn't have to work or worry about what other people thought today, what would I most love to do?' Now think about how you can give yourself 10 per cent of that today.

Wow, I can have two days off when I bleed and not feel guilty. It's OK not to run on the day I bleed, and I have an excuse to go to bed at 9 pm. It helps me to care for my more vulnerable parts and it's nice to sit with that and dream.

CASSIE, 24

Usually women just want to do nothing except curl up with a good book or a pile of magazines and not have to worry about anything. Look at your schedule. Be ruthless about cutting out what's absolutely not essential, such as that lunch date with your friend. Watch how you leak energy by getting caught up in dramas or gossip or having to listen to someone's problems. Excuse yourself from these situations as quickly as possible. It's the day when *you* need to receive. And remember to eat well! The more you sustain this awareness, the more you'll find you can make little changes that will open this renewal phase for you and the more effective and authoritative you'll be in your professional life.

Regardless of whether or not you suffer with your periods, you might come to regard time out at your period as an important part of your lifestyle along with exercise and a good diet for maintaining your health. Once you taste the benefits of this time you'll have no difficulty taking time out for yourself in the future. Initially it might only be half an hour, but more begets more, and just like when you eat chocolate, it can become a rather delicious addiction. And it's simply good medicine to take this time each month—for menstruation that is, not chocolate!

Your natural calm tips

1. Keep track of where you are in your cycle. This will be one of your basic calm-building practices. Mark in your diary the day menstruation is roughly due. If your cycle is very regular then just marking that in the diary can be enough.

2. Reduce commitments around your period. Do only what you have to, and reduce that again! No-one has to know why you're not so available. You can write in your diary 'PLAY date with myself'.

3. Make sure you have some good food in the house so that you don't end up rushing out to do a 'big shop' or eat junk. Both will undermine your calm.

4. Be prepared so that you're not pressured.

5. Move slowly at the pace of your body and mood rather than your head, which is generally more driven and speedy.

6. Have some 'nothing' time to cruise, rest, dream, wander aimlessly and do something just for yourself. Aim for this to be as close to the first day of bleeding as possible.

CHAPTER 25

GETTING HIGH . . . NATURALLY

The first time I came off the Pill people asked me what drug was making me so happy! I felt energetic and really positive.

KIM, 37

One way or another we all want to enjoy more heightened states of feeling and awareness. For some it may be through rave parties, drugs, drinking, obsessive exercise or sex, or for others, through tai chi, meditation or yoga. Yet, as women, we have an amazing opportunity each month to experience states that can range from exquisite, heart-opening love to ecstasy. Yep, your period is a natural high, and it's free and legal. However, you do need to create the physical and emotional space for the good feelings to unfold, which does require some effort on your part.

Creating the physical space means taking the time to be alone and filtering out unnecessary external stimulation. Creating the emotional space involves respecting your feelings—not fighting them, but truly 'giving in' to what you're actually experiencing and, above all, letting yourself be vulnerable.

The gift of vulnerability

One of the reasons many women struggle with the cycle is *because* of a sense of loss of control, and feeling vulnerable leading into menstruation. Your emotions may seem to have a life of their own. However, while vulnerability can feel like a weakness, without it it's hard to know yourself. As psychologists Doctors Hal and Sidra Stone remind us, 'If we have no access to our vulnerability we do not know *who* we are, *what* we like, and what we *don't* like, we do not know what makes us feel *good* and what makes us feel *bad*' [emphasis in original].[1]

Love, intimacy and ecstasy can *only* come from a place of openness and vulnerability. When you start to feel less 'together' and more sensitive as you get close to bleeding, which we often label PMS, it's your very own preparation for accessing these glorious feelings. So allow yourself to feel tender and vulnerable so you can access the feelings of love and ecstasy that await you as you bleed. During her period Billi feels ecstatic—like her whole being is singing and everything feels 'right' in her. It can be quite intoxicating, and she seriously wonders what drug she's on sometimes!

Accessing your inner bliss

When you start to experience any of that PMS stuff of doubting yourself, feeling overwhelmed, irritable, or not wanting to go out or engage with people, you know you are preparing for your natural high.

During the 24 to 48 hours before bleeding, depending on your character and outer circumstances, there can sometimes be an exquisitely tender and open moment in which your senses are completely alive to the smallest nuance. If you can slow down and enter this place consciously, you may experience stillness (that natural calm) and the feelings of love. You may not necessarily experience this every month. The main instruction is to follow and give validity to what *you* experience, and let that reveal its hidden riches.

As the blood starts to flow, there's a release, a natural high. The cycle has begun its upward arc and you are reborn. Naturally women's experience will differ on this, but the longer you pause and the more rested you are, the more pleasures will open to you—pleasures of ease and softness or feelings of excitement and charge.

One woman plays her best netball on the first day of her period—she's obviously experiencing that great charge. Another suddenly feels she can run further on the first day of bleeding. Interestingly, although you can get a sudden burst of energy, it's wise not to dissipate it on lots of activity. Simply let it circulate through you and re-energise your body and spirit instead, and then you can enjoy all that creative inspiration.

The vulnerability before bleeding can, on the other hand, expose you to bits of yourself you don't like. You may experience self-doubt, despair, high anxiety or being out of control, which can be acted out in excessive drinking, using drugs, or through other addictive behaviours. If this happens you may be a highly sensitive and intuitive person and don't yet know how to handle it. Try some of the suggestions outlined in Chapter 22 'Your very own feedback loop' and Chapter 23 'Tapping your intuition'.

Understanding ecstasy

Ecstasy is a big concept as Jalaja Bonheim reminds us in her book *The Hunger for Ecstasy*. It's 'intense and outrageous . . . [and] blows our minds open to a reality that is wild, beautiful, loving, abundant beyond our wildest dreams'.[2] It's a gift that we make room for and not something we ourselves can create. When you have a degree of ease in your own skin—relishing the sensuality of your body and the pulsing of the life force—you're opening the 'ecstasy door', and that includes the doorway to sexual ecstasy.

> The best news is that the female body is designed for ecstasy.

Menstruation is like lovemaking, birthing and meditation. All require quiet, space, dimmed light, the ability to go deep inside and a capacity to let go in order to truly enter the ecstasy. Placing yourself in beautiful surroundings or being out in nature can also enhance the experience. Menstruation does the rest for you.

The best news is that the female body is designed for ecstasy. Diana Richardson, author of *Tantric Orgasm for Women*, outlines the capacity of women for ecstasy during lovemaking that opens the way for men too. Dr Sarah Buckley, author of *Gentle Birth, Gentle Mothering*, writes about ecstasy as an intrinsic part of the birth process—'every woman's genetic blueprint'.[3] When we are given drugs such as the Pill or those used during birth (some of which may, of course, be necessary), this ecstatic potential is interrupted. The more it's interrupted, the more we may find ourselves relying on outer sources for our 'high' and not trusting the wisdom and power of our own bodies.

If you're grounded in your cycle, then you've also taken steps towards experiencing greater sexual pleasure and being better prepared for the journey of pregnancy and the ecstasy of birth.

Reconnection

The high of menstruation comes from letting go and reconnecting to your deeper self. Think of it like coming home after the end of a full-on day of work. As you chill out, you start to come back to life again and your mood lifts. At your period you get a highly amplified version of this.

Strangely, when you 'come home' to yourself you also connect with a feeling of something much bigger than you; a sense of belonging and meaningfulness that comes when you feel your place in the big scheme of things. It's as though you're plugged back in to the centre of the Cosmos.

> Valuing your cycle will give you access to a greater inner aliveness.

In shutting down the cycle, the Pill, for all its apparent power to free us sexually, economically and politically, deadens your wonderful inbuilt facility for creative and spiritual renewal. Valuing your cycle will give you access to a greater inner aliveness, the world will feel more magical and meaningful, your intuitive and psychic radar will be humming and you'll feel greater peace and self-acceptance.

CHAPTER 26

PERIOD POWER AND HOW TO GET MORE OF IT

*I would have ended up burnt out and bitter if
I hadn't discovered the power of the cycle.*

EMMA, 29

Emma is an ambitious, determined and outspoken woman who doesn't let much stand in her path. Her periods always seemed like an unnecessary obstacle to her. As director of her own highly successful personal training company, she also had a demanding fitness training program which was probably why she hadn't had a period for seven years, but she wasn't unhappy with that state of affairs.

When she attended Alexandra's *Women Power and the Body* course, her period suddenly started to flow after only two hours—not something she was expecting at all. It seemed almost miraculous. Discovering the cycle, for Emma, was like she had been given a map that helped to explain all the disparate bits of information she had observed about women.

As she said, 'I would have ended up burnt out and bitter if I hadn't discovered the power of the cycle.'

What is period power?

Periods have had some lousy press over the last few thousand years. They've apparently made us unclean, dumb, weak, bad, mad, dangerous or just plain difficult, and have been used as a reason to deny us education and political, economic and spiritual power. Even today, despite relatively good health education most women are still embarrassed about it and, unlike sex, it's still not a topic for comfortable public discussion.

For periods to have accrued so much negativity, one thing that you can be assured of is that something *very* interesting, even powerful, has to be going on. We've explored how the cycle gives you feedback about your physical and mental health and gets you in touch with your natural inbuilt de-stressing zone. It also opens you to a secret knowledge source inside yourself and can give you a dose of ecstasy or feeling just plain high each month. That's all power. Without having to meditate (although that's also great to do and can enhance your menstrual experience), you can begin to enjoy quite blissful, centred, calm states just by being very aware of these natural powers.

> For menstruation to have accrued so much negativity, one thing that you can be assured of is that something very interesting, even powerful, has to be going on.

The menstrual cycle acts as your inner creative compass—an inherent smartness in your being that you can leverage to create real success and wellbeing. It's a bit like having your own personal coach guiding and inspiring you. This is period power.

When you're in touch with period power you know what's right and not right for you. You feel confident, sexy and comfortable with yourself. You know how to harness your inner energies for optimum success. And you're not afraid to be vulnerable, because you know that's the secret key to the most exquisite intimacy with yourself and with your partner.

How to access your period power

Throughout the book we've been encouraging you to chart your cycle as a basic self-care practice. The cycle is like a map for exploring different states of being, thinking and feeling that can help you to be more creative, powerful and happy. To fully access your period power you need to be aware of the inner seasons of your body.

The first part of the cycle, the days after you've finished bleeding, is your inner spring—*a new beginning*. As with spring, there's a feeling of enthusiasm, freshness and renewed vigour, followed by the wonderful ripeness and out-there-ness of ovulation, a time when you may feel more easy and relaxed with the world. This is the summer of your cycle—the *having it all* phase. And just as the seasons turn and the light shifts, so your mood shifts to a different perspective in the premenstrual phase. Autumn can bring more reflection and stirring of deeper feelings, so the latter part of the menstrual cycle also brings greater depth of feeling and shifts in energy. This is when you *get real* with yourself and what you're doing in your life—your feedback time.

Finally menstruation, the wintertime of your cycle, comes round and you might want to be more withdrawn and quieter as one tends to be in winter. This is the classic *chill out* phase of any creative endeavour and that includes your life. You know—it's the moment when you just have to walk away from what you're working on for a while because you're over it . . . momentarily!

Each phase of the creative process is necessary for making your goals happen. If you try to skip one, and usually it's the 'getting real' phase, you may find yourself treading water in your life, never really having a sense of completing anything properly. Homoeopath Alastair Gray has observed in his years of practice that women taking the Pill, and therefore being cut off from their menstrual map, can seem dull and directionless.

A new beginning

While the first day of bleeding is considered as day one of your menstrual cycle, and certainly menstruation can bring a real sense of release and relief, you're still in the chill-out zone. Your new beginning phase really gets going once the blood has eased. You'll know the moment—you'll feel clearer and lighter.

Experiencing more clarity about your direction, a new beginning is a natural time for initiating ideas and plans, whether it's for the coming month or longer term. You may also have had some inspirations as you were bleeding some of which you might want to activate this month. Remember, your period is your classic window of opportunity moment in which creative inspirations can burst through.

The power of this time lies in feeling fresh, free and relatively unencumbered. It's as though the menstrual bleed has cleared out a lot of old 'stuff' and you can start over with your life with renewed enthusiasm. Anything feels possible now, but even as you're re-energised and want to get out there, be a little self-contained. Your freshness of spirit has a certain delicacy, an innocence that needs to be cherished. Ease yourself gently back into the full flow of life.

Set clear goals for the coming month, or reaffirm current ones. Write them in a

> The menstrual cycle acts as your inner creative compass—an inherent smartness in your being that you can leverage to create real success and well-being.

journal or have a board on which you pin up words or images of your goals, and include a picture of yourself in the centre.

If you have a recurring emotional reactivity in the getting real phase, that PMS stuff, resolve this month to address that issue rather than just getting cranky and irritable about it every month. For instance, if you and your boyfriend end up having the same argument, now you've got the energy to address the issue.

Take a moment to centre yourself: close your eyes, focus on the in and out of your breath and, when you feel a little stilled, make a definite statement about what you are choosing for this month: 'This month I'm choosing to . . . (fill in here what you want to do, create or address)'. There's a real potency in making a clear statement like this, especially if you speak it out loud, though you might want to be alone to do that. You have added power now to 'charge up' your dreams, so capitalise on this energy.

I'm excited in that beginning phase of the cycle but I feel precarious too, like how I feel after a holiday or after making my New Year's resolutions.

AMY, 37

Billi loves waiting for the clarity of this phase to grab her. It's like a big 'Yes' from her being to go for some specific thing that month. She'll write notes in her journal and then revisit her notes at the end of the menstrual month to see how she went.

Strangely, some women can experience a drop in energy, even depression in this early phase of the cycle, the very opposite of what we've discussed here. When that's the case it may mean you're rundown, pushing yourself too much, haven't given yourself sufficient rest at menstruation, or have a chronic health problem that's depleting you. This is more feedback. Being more in gear with the different phases of the cycle, getting plenty of rest, improving your diet and utilising the skills of a holistic health practitioner can start to turn this around.

Barbara feels so alive and charged when she bleeds that the new beginning phase can initially feel like an anticlimax—almost a feeling of grief—as she leaves behind those heightened feelings. This is normal and does pass as the momentum of the new cycle takes hold.

Having it all

You're in superwoman territory now. Just as your cycle peaks at ovulation, you're at a peak of drive and activity. Conservation of your energy won't be at the top of your list because you have energy to burn. Having it all can feel possible and you're out doing all you can to manifest your goals.

> *I have a big energy in me around ovulation, a real charge that I have to use.*
> *I'm like a captain steering a ship . . . and have lots of pots on the boil . . . it's so*
> *highly productive. I love it.*
>
> AMY, 37

This is classically the time of easy flow and networking, where you can be all things to all people, be accepting of others and life, and not overly challenging of the status quo. You'll probably feel pretty good in your own skin, attractive and even a magnet, drawing things and people to you. Nothing feels too much. You can overstuff your schedule and pretty much get away with it and even multi-task in your sleep!

If you've taken time in the new beginning phase to focus on your goals, you'll find you can really leverage this phase to the max, ticking lots of things off on your 'to do' list. However, if you're a bit directionless you could squander your energy and even feel somewhat empty and unsettled. Equally, you may just want to enjoy being out having an easy, playful time. It's simply about being in touch with what's important to you at any one moment, and making clear choices.

Use this time to ask for that pay rise you've been wanting, for experimenting with new activities, working opportunities, testing new ideas or addressing those issues that always bug you with your partner or friends. You'll be able to do it with more delicacy and care for the other person at this time.

Some women can feel a sudden down moment soon after ovulating, and while there might be any number of reasons for this, one thing to consider is a lack of a sense of any real achievement happening in your life overall, a lack of 'birthing' something.

> Connecting to the deeper knowledge of your body through the cycle is like opening to a secret power source.

Kyra is quite challenged by the ovulatory phase, experiencing feelings similar to PMS angst. Working freelance for some time in the film industry has lost its shine, and she doesn't feel it's her thing anymore. But what is? She doesn't know. And to top it off she'd like to have children but the timing isn't right. Kyra has an ambitious drive but nowhere to put it. As she comes in to ovulation there's an urgent feeling of 'must conceive NOW', as though her body is strongly speaking about her yearning for an actual baby and her spirit is demanding creative avenues to express itself. Once ovulation has passed she's feels that she's lost something—'an egg, of course, a baby chance. I'm a woman who knows how to separate my head thoughts from my heart feelings,' she said. 'I can see that this is my body talking to me, not my head, giving me real insight into myself.'

If you're a woman who wants to have a child and are not in a position to, or are struggling to conceive, the post-ovulatory moment can bring grief as the chance of conceiving has passed for that month.

Getting real

If you want to 'have it all' then you need to get real with yourself. Superwoman can spread herself too thinly and start to run out of energy. An overstuffed schedule can start to look like a nightmare, so now it's time to re-examine your priorities.

As a wife, mother and owner of a small business, Alicia can easily overdo it if she's not thoughtful. Many a time she's caught herself out happily booking up her schedule when she's in her having it all phase, forgetting that when she arrives at the getting real time that she isn't going to be able to do it all, because she's human after all. The penny is finally dropping. Now she marks the getting real time in her diary so that she won't run herself ragged.

> If you want to 'have it all' then you need to get real with yourself.

In this phase you can learn about what is and isn't working in your life. Remember, it's 'feedback time'—the time when you need to care for and assert yourself more clearly, establish stronger boundaries and experience a greater drive to clear away obstacles that are stalling your growth. You'll know this moment. Your sunny disposition won't be quite so sunny or harmonious, and you might feel more of an 'edge' in you.

Your menstrual cycle is pulling you inwards to focus on your core purpose. Shemiran described it as like coming back into her body. When you come back into your body you really connect to your true feelings. It's the great reality check moment. In any business endeavour there's a lot of behind-the-scenes work that makes the business possible. The getting real phase is the natural behind-the-scenes time for both the business of you and your literal business.

It's not the glamorous phase of any creative endeavour. Now you must examine whether your ideas work, if they're good enough, what needs to change, how you can improve them and so on. You may find yourself asking similar questions about your own life. Is what I'm doing right for me? Does anything need to be altered or changed or trimmed back? Or perhaps everything is just fine but you have to stand back from what you're doing to get another perspective. You have a more detached power that can be critical, punchy and incisive and allows you to edit, refine, cut back, sort out and clean up. It's not unlike pruning plants to support the regrowth in the next season. Without proper pruning, the new growth would be undermined. And interestingly, many women literally find themselves doing a big clean-out just before they bleed.

The nice, polite, socialised self in you bites the dust now and out leaps your inner powerbroker. Sometimes known as the Bitch, or Babe in Total Control of Herself, this feisty, assertive, provocative energy can allow you to have those 'difficult' conversations and challenge the status quo. With your capacity to cut through the crap to the core issue you'll be unstoppable, but you do need to be mindful of how you can polarise people more easily. This isn't necessarily bad—it can be very creative—but don't expect people to like you for being so direct. However, the more accepting you are of this provocative energy, the more skilled you can become in using it.

Helen deliberately uses this time to take on challenging situations or people at work because she feels so empowered and less fazed about others' reactions. Francis, who was involved in a protracted legal conflict, always seemed to sit down to tackle the issue in the getting real phase. She did it quite unconsciously, as though she instinctively knew she had a more gutsy authority to handle the difficult tensions. Susannah simply doesn't pull her punches anymore in the workplace. Blessed with a more penetrating insight, she speaks her mind on what's working or not working. Of course some are uncomfortable being challenged, but because Susannah likes her assertive intelligence, she's able to use it congruently and wisely.

If you've had hurtful or painful experiences to handle in the past, remember that you could find this getting real phase stirs all this up or just leaves you feeling pretty yuk. If this is the case, plan ahead to give yourself a special pampering treat, or line up a good friend to hang out with. The simple act of charting your cycle can help

> The nice, polite, socialised self in you bites the dust now and out leaps your inner powerbroker.

you be more accepting of yourself and more able to negotiate this trouble spot. You can also try writing your feelings in your journal.

The getting real phase is the time to work smarter not harder, becoming more grounded and realistic about how to use your time and energy. And as it's also about tidying up and completions, it's a good idea wherever possible to hold off starting something new or making any big decisions until after you've bled. It's not that you can't do those things at this time, but rather there's an extra magic, that natural wave of enthusiasm and clarity, to capitalise on at the beginning of the cycle that you can take advantage of. It's like the gardener or the farmer following Nature's seasons for planting and harvesting.

> The getting real phase is the time to work smarter not harder, becoming more grounded and realistic about how to use your time and energy.

We can sometimes 'lose it' at this time. Remember not to dismiss your reactivity as 'just premenstrual'. Apologise for *how* you spoke if you need to but stand by what you said. This is strong energy and it takes some years of living to use wisely. And it will be stronger for some than others because of their overall temperament. The more comfortable you are with yourself, the easier it will be to channel this force.

Chilling out

One of the things you may notice in the last days of the cycle as you draw into your period is the desire to slow down and do less. You might feel you want to drop your bundle and walk off into the sunset, leaving all your cares behind you. Or you feel a bit more vulnerable, tender and dreamy. This is a sign that you're entering chill-out time—your window of opportunity that opens you to a sense of renewal. Lydia can suffer from quite bad PMS mood swings but notices that they suddenly ease 24 to 48 hours before her period. That's her signal that she's arrived at her chill-out zone.

*I was giving and fighting and nothing was coming back in, but the battle just
fell away once I knew about the cycle . . . I never understood forgiveness
before but now I can.*

EMMA, 29

When you sense any of those signals, slow down if you can. This is the utter still point of the cycle; it's the moment not for pushing any agendas but rather for letting go and being gentle and sweet with yourself. The more you can do that, the more you'll open a door inside yourself to feelings of love and self-acceptance. And then, as the blood flows, come the ideas, inspirations and that wonderful upsurge of energy we spoke of in the previous chapter. Your creativity is renewed and you feel refreshed. The new cycle has begun and you'll come to your work with different eyes—problems may seem less like problems or, surprisingly, will solve themselves without you doing anything. As you speak from this place you can assert yourself without polarising people and you may find that others really listen. That's the gift of your body each month as you bleed.

Even though you might feel reinvigorated, now is the time to burn the 'to do' list and just hang out and be with yourself, perhaps recording your thoughts in a journal, or letting them gestate quietly inside. Give yourself the experience of *no pressure at all*. Being in 'doing' mode will block the creative inspiration from flowing. And when you can really let go, you repair and mend and can go out freshly minted to start a whole new cycle of activity and manifestation.

With your intuitive and instinctual powers now at their height, use this visionary time to tap in to your inner wisdom for insights on all aspects of your life, feel into your emotional depths and love what you see there. Light a candle to yourself and imagine you are being anointed by a sacred blessing from the Great Goddess herself, saying, 'You are beautiful, gorgeous, and perfect just as you are'. Do that every month as you bleed and feel your self-esteem quietly blossom.

> Kirrilee would really allow herself to empty out by getting a large sheet of paper and pouring out all the emotional stuff going on in her life. When she had finished she would then draw and write all she wanted in her life, giving herself compliments and drawing positive images.

Think of the first half of the cycle as going out to meet the world and the second half as returning home to connect with yourself. The having it all phase is about giving out and the chill-out phase is about receiving. While we appreciate growth and activity, we're generally not very good at letting go, being with ourselves and letting others give to us. If you want to feel stronger and more complete as a person you do need to integrate the doing and the being, the giving and the receiving. The cycle simply reminds you of all that.

You will of course have your own unique take on the cycle that is connected to your temperament, personal ambitions, overall health and the environments you work and live in, as well as whether or not you're in a relationship, have children and your general level of confidence. We've outlined the seasons of your cycle as a template that you can use as a starting place to discover the full character of your own menstrual map. Above all, trust what you sense and feel unfolding in your own body.

Opening to a secret power source

Each period is like opening a new present . . . I tell women now that they are the greatest untapped energy source.
EMMA, 29

Connecting to the deeper knowledge of your body through the cycle is like opening up to a secret power source. When she reflects back Meghan feels betrayed at being kept from this knowledge when the Pill was the only option offered her for contraception. Learning about how her menstrual cycle works has been a deeply pleasurable experience, helping to awaken in her the pleasure of being herself.

Now that her cycle is back, she's enjoying the natural currents of energy, sometimes out there and connecting with others and at other times needing her private space and time. She recognises how critical this is for achieving things in the world. She's learnt to ask for what she needs, and being more aware of her needs and how they change has made her more tolerant of others' shifting moods and demands. It's also changed the way she deals with conflict. Now she feels more empowered to say 'I'm uncomfortable with this', or 'I'm feeling that' and dealing with the issue in a much more proactive way.

Emma has been radically changed by this process. Not only has incorporation of this smart approach to the cycle into all her personal training programs proved very successful, she has felt transformed. 'My intuition has really come alive. I've attracted so much more business,' she said. While Emma had an enormous capacity for pushing through any blocks or challenges she encountered, this was building hardness and bitterness in her. But when her period returned she felt the resistance fall away, and compassion and grace flood her being. 'I was giving and fighting and nothing was coming back in, but the battle just fell away once I knew about the cycle . . . I never understood forgiveness before but now I can,' she said. 'Each period is like opening a new present . . . I tell women now that they are the greatest untapped energy source.'

CHAPTER 27

THE NATURAL WAY TO MENSTRUAL WELLBEING

We don't, as a society, give intrinsic value to fertility as a sign of health, of wholeness, of wellbeing, of a body doing OK. We are creating huge problems with this attitude, for individuals and society as a whole.

WENDY DUMARESQ, HERBALIST

Getting menstrual health counselling was Penny's last resort before trying the Pill. At 26 she'd been experiencing very painful periods and nausea, often spending the first two days in bed. She was resentful that this 'affliction' was getting in the way of the rest of her life, particularly her triathlon training. Sometimes she'd drag herself along to an early morning session doped up on painkillers just to prove that she wasn't lazy or weak.

Through counselling she learnt to see how her excessive training (between two and six hours a day) premenstrually was depleting her energy. She was encouraged to stop resisting her natural cycle of tiredness and to give herself permission to be restful and nurturing, and encouraged to structure her training program around her menstrual cycle. It's interesting to note that the general notion of 'recovery time' is being increasingly recognised as an important aspect of athletic training.

To treat her symptoms, Penny got acupuncture and attended to her diet, cooking delicious, organic meals. She still gets frustrated with her body and challenged by feelings of failure. However, in spite of this when she asks herself, 'Could I go back to the way things were?', the answer from deep inside her is that 'Life is much richer and more exciting now'.

If you suffer with menstrual problems, accessing all the wonderful attributes of period power may feel like a distant dream. However, as you begin to respect menstruation as *potentially* a really good thing, something will shift inside you that will indeed help you to heal, as it did for Penny.

Menstrual health tip 1—doing what you love
If you didn't have to worry about the rest of the world when you bleed, what would you most love to be doing? Find a way to do at least 10 per cent of that.

The new approach to your health

Our new approach to menstrual wellbeing is based on respect for the real intelligence of your cycle. The old way which viewed the menstrual cycle itself as the problem is very last century and counterproductive to your health. When you cooperate with your own rhythm and needs this builds confidence and eases tension, which in turn alleviates symptoms. In the long term doing this *as much as you can* within the demands of work and life commitments is the way to go. For some the results can be quite radical.

After learning about period power, Meredith's menstrual pain lifted: 'I'm experiencing a totally pain-free bleed for the first time in fourteen or more years. Since the workshop I seem to experience my cycle in glorious slow motion, which serves to amplify the changes in tempo.'

Clare has experienced a slow revolution over a year. She used to experience intense period pains, hot and cold sweats and wanted to do nothing but curl up during the first two days of bleeding. But since she began listening to her cycle each month and created a safe and nurturing environment when her period came, things have changed dramatically. Her pain has almost gone and she doesn't have the sweats anymore. In her words, 'I can fully embrace the depths, which are luscious, creative and sacred. It's a time I look forward to now'.

This we cannot forget . . . a woman cannot expect to have a healthy menstrual cycle, if she's not feeling emotionally balanced. The two worlds are connected. This has long been recognised by Eastern traditions such as Traditional Chinese Medicine and Ayurveda.
ANGELA HYWOOD, NATUROPATH

Seven steps to feeling fabulous
- Begin to access your period power.
- Eat a diet of natural, whole, fresh foods.
- Get plenty of good quality rest and repair time, especially at menstruation.
- Reduce the load of toxins in your environment.
- Enjoy a sustainable exercise program that includes time outdoors to give you regular doses of natural light for Vitamin D.
- Visit a holistic health practitioner for a healing program tailor made for you.
- Maintain patience and kindness towards yourself.

The joy of real food

Food is about pleasure, sharing and nourishment. Good food is also marvellous for healing all menstrual problems. The good news for you is that healthy food can be delicious and not some kind of punishment or deprivation.

For many women food is not emotionally neutral. It would be rare to find one of us who hasn't had any angst over weight and food at some point in our lives. So it's important to approach this topic gently and kindly. Unless you're a person who likes to jump into the deep end of dietary change, we encourage you to make small steps that are sustainable, adding more over time. As you get used to the changes and feel the benefits, you'll probably start to find you have an increasing aversion to junk foods.

> **Menstrual health tip 2—lemon water**
> To assist your liver and aid digestion take a couple of lemons, ideally organic, scrub well, roughly chop up and place in a glass container (it must be glass). Add 2–3 cups of purified water and let it stand for at least 3 hours in the fridge. Enjoy drinking any time you like but especially first thing in the morning and before and after meals.

Sandra has followed a healthy eating program over a number of years, slowly stopping unsupportive foods when she felt ready. Today she's still able to maintain this healthy program and, more importantly, her 'period pain from hell' has gone. Now she just experiences some tenderness and a little minor cramping as her blood starts to flow, which for her is just miraculous.

Julia, on the other hand, is one of those women who can jump into the deep end of change. Suffering from endometriosis, she took on the healing diet with gusto and within three months her period pain had gone. Whether she can sustain this over time, given the pressures of her high-powered job, she doesn't know yet, but it does speak of the enormous power of food to heal.

Falling off the wagon of good eating is only human. It happens—simply get back on as soon as you can. Even plan for breakouts if you're struggling, but make them in the first half of your cycle as much as possible, though we do appreciate you may have a PMS binge moment of sweet, chocolatey, oily, rich things! The more you plan for 'those' moments the less junk you'll probably eat. And the more nourished you are, the less you'll crave the foods that are not healthy. A naturopath can also help you with specific supplements to deal with sugar cravings.

You can have the best diet in the world but still may not be absorbing your nutrients. This can happen if your digestion is poor, or if you have food allergies, candida or irritable bowel syndrome. Women with menstrual problems may often suffer from digestive troubles and we'd recommend you get professional support to deal with this. Period pain and PMS can improve markedly.

Allow at least three months for your new diet to take effect. Leading into and during menstruation follow the food 'rules' as closely as you can and aim to eat light, easily digestible meals around your period to minimise PMS and pain. Above all, be prepared for menstruation by having good food in the house ahead of time so that you don't have to shop when you're feeling unwell or overtired.

Menstrual health tip 3—nettle tea
For a mineral rich tonic that nourishes and stabilises energy in the reproductive/hormonal system, promotes healthy bones, helps ease cramping and profuse menstrual flow, and is a great pick-me-up and general all-round ally for women, place two teaspoons of loose dried organic nettles in a jar and top up with one and a half cups of filtered water. Let stand overnight. Drink at room temperature or heat up (without boiling) for a hot drink. You can also make it like a normal tea although you won't get the full blast of nutrients.

In the health industry there are debates on what constitutes a good diet. On top of this we all have different nutritional needs. However, there are certain things that we can all agree on and that is the quality of the food: how it is grown and prepared. Highly processed and junk food is dead food. The life force is beaten out of it along with most of its essential nutrients. On top of that they include ingredients that are bad for you such as additives, colourings, genetically modified ingredients, hydrogenated oils and the residue of chemicals used to remove things such as fat in 'fat free' foods, or to process flour so that it will have a longer shelf life.

When we refer to processed food we're referring to food that has been refined using high tech methods. Traditional slow forms of processing such as fermenting, drying, pickling and cooking are fine as long as, of course, no chemical additives have been introduced, which they usually are in many commercial products. Read labels very carefully.

Organic or biodynamic food is the most nourishing, however, if you're not able to access or afford this, eating fresh food, as opposed to processed or junk food, still means you're way ahead. Real food is fresh and whole. Genetically modified food is not. Nor is margarine, including even the so-called 'healthy' margarines.

The following is a guide to what is best to eat and what to avoid.[1] When you see a holistic health practitioner they may fine-tune this outline to better suit your specific needs. You'll notice coffee, tea and chocolate on the 'to avoid' list. This might feel a bit much at first. If you feel you must drink coffee have the real thing, fresh and not instant. If you must eat chocolate, buy good quality organic brands.

The *really enjoyable* good food guide
- Real food—fresh and whole.
- Lots of vegetables (including some seaweed) and some fruit.
- Whole grains, legumes and fresh nuts.
- If you eat animal products, consume meat, dairy foods and eggs only from pasture-fed, ideally organic, animals.

- Some raw food—including raw milk if you're lucky enough to find it.
- Eat fermented foods regularly, like yoghurt, sauerkraut and pickles.
- Use traditional cold pressed vegetable oils only.
- Use filtered water for cooking and drinking.
- Use natural sugars in moderation, like raw honey, maple syrup, date sugar, dehydrated cane sugar juice (Rapadura) and stevia powder.

The *not* good food guide—to be avoided
- Soft drinks.
- Artificial sweeteners including sucrulose and aspartame.
- Commercially processed foods.
- Soy products produced in non-traditional ways.
- Coffee, tea and chocolate.
- Hydrogenated fats and oils.
- Excessive amounts of processed grain, like pasta, bread, cakes and biscuits.
- All refined vegetable oils, including soy, corn, safflower, canola or cottonseed.
- Processed, pasteurised, ultra-pasteurised, low-fat, skim milk, powdered milk or imitation milk products.
- Battery-produced eggs and factory farmed meat and fish.
- Highly processed luncheon meat and sausages.
- Quick-rise breads and extruded breakfast cereals.
- Canned, waxed and irradiated fruits and vegetables.
- Genetically modified foods.
- Artificial food additives and colourings.

Menstrual health tip 4—miso soup

Like the ubiquitous chicken soup, miso soup is a panacea for all ills. Nourishing and alkalising, for those of you who live life on the run it's also quick and easy to prepare. For an instant pick-me-up put approximately half a teaspoon of miso in a cup add some hot water, chopped shallots and freshly grated ginger. Or, throw a handful of vegetables (eg Chinese greens, white radish, pumpkin, green beans) in a pot with enough water for a bowl of soup. Add some seaweed such as kombu or wakame for extra minerals and bring to the boil. Simmer until vegetables are soft. Place miso in your soup bowl and add some liquid to make a paste, and then add the boiled vegetables and remaining liquid. Avoid boiling the miso because it kills the friendly lactobacillus that aids your digestion.

Rest is radical

In the West we have an epidemic of exhaustion. We push, push, push and don't allow for enough downtime. We could all do with more rest. For women menstruation is the natural time for this and as a bonus you'll get some of that 'natural calm'.

Slow down as you come into and during menstruation. Go to bed earlier. Apart from getting good quality rest, there's evidence that the extra dreaming time is good for easing PMS.[2] It's the all-round number one remedy *and* it costs nothing. Rachel found this approach very effective for her period pain. Instead of taking painkillers and continuing to keep going as she would usually do, she decided to really let go and rest. Her pain was greatly reduced and as a bonus she got lots of real insights into herself that made her rethink some of the things she was doing in her life—she was getting in touch with her inner wisdom.

Exercise

A regular movement program does all sorts of wonderful things for
you, including lifting your mood. And it really works for menstrual
problems too. Find ways to build exercise into your life that is workable
and pleasurable. Practise incidental exercise such as climbing the stairs
at work rather than taking the lift as well as heading for that gym or
yoga class.

Some menstrual symptoms are connected with structural problems
in the body. If you work all day in an office hunched over a computer this
will affect the structure of your body and the functioning of your organs.
Regular stretching, exercise, a massage or a visit to the chiropractor or
osteopath can work wonders for healing menstrual problems, particularly
period pain.

Practices such as yoga, tai chi, qi gong, and Feldenkrais build an
inner calmness even as you exercise. And your teacher may also be able to
recommend specific movements or poses that strengthen your endocrine
system and pelvic region.

Make sure you get twenty minutes outside daily, if possible, to get
your vitamin D from natural light. Before 9 am in the southern hemisphere and between 8 am and 8 pm in daylight hours in the northern
hemisphere are the optimum times.

Cleaning up your environment

Many menstrual problems are linked to increasing environmental pollution, whether it's from the products you use on your body, in your food and water, the everyday chemicals you use to clean your house, plastics and other synthetic material, or pollution from transport, industry and agribusiness farming. The accumulative effect of all these environmental stressors plays havoc with your immune system, and therefore your body's ability to repair itself.

I have a sense that the really beneficial changes were detoxifying my home and body products, and prioritising rest during the 'winter' aspect of the cycle.

ANNALISE, 28

Use plant-based beauty products rather than petrochemically based ones. A list of some natural ingredients doesn't mean a product is completely natural. Read labels carefully and question all ingredients. There are a number of companies today producing high quality products—you can research these online and at your local health food store.

Use a water filter and buy organic and biodynamic food according to availability and your budget. Find friendly cleaning agents at your health food store or alternatively stick to the old fashioned methods of bicarbonate of soda and vinegar.

Technology is wonderful—who'd want to be without it? But there's a shadow side in the form of the electromagnetic radiation. This is emitted by microwave ovens, televisions, computers and mobile phones as well as by other electrical devices—even seemingly harmless appliances like hairdryers and electric clocks. We're also exposed to radiation when we have X-rays, are near high voltage power lines and when we fly in aeroplanes. Do be thoughtful about this. The official UK Health Protection Agency has acknowledged in a report that electro sensitivity is a genuine health condition.[3] You may be more sensitive than others, especially during your 'getting real' time, making you overly 'wired' and thus interfering with your ability to access natural calm and enjoy heightened intuition around your period.

Find ways to give yourself a break from technology. Simply being out in nature is one obvious way. You could also try nights without television or being on the computer, especially if you've been on the latter all day at work. Keep your conversations on mobiles very brief and don't use microwave ovens. Avoid Wi-Fi technology—there are real concerns being expressed in the UK and Europe now on the hazards of this technology for everyone's wellbeing.[4] Avoid computers and televisions in the bedroom but if you have no alternative, make sure they're unplugged from the socket every night.

> **Menstrual health tip 6—Epsom salts bath**
> An excellent de-stressor, the magnesium in Epsom salts is an essential mineral for easing menstrual woes, including PMS, cramping and endometriosis. It also helps to oxygenate the body, release toxins and is particularly beneficial if you're exposed to a lot of electromagnetic radiation, for example from computers. Add four to six cups of Epsom salts to a comfortably hot bath (enough that you sweat a bit) and luxuriate in it for twenty minutes. Don't shower afterwards. Lie flat for ten minutes wrapped in towels to maintain your body heat and let yourself deeply relax.

Enjoy the process

Healing will take you on a journey involving change that can be exhilarating and sometimes challenging. Healing focuses on building your overall wellbeing and not just on suppression of your symptoms. Healing involves your body, mind and spirit as an integrated whole. Because of this, healing can include such diverse strategies as changing your job so that you feel happier, addressing some emotional issues, perhaps in counselling, getting out of an unsupportive relationship as well as the obvious practices of good diet and other natural remedies that we've mentioned.

I really love my new job. And that's certainly affecting my PMS for the better.
FRAN, 32

Healing involves noticing small day-to-day shifts and changes as they slowly add up to a deep and sustained sense of wellbeing.

You may also need more concentrated remedies to supplement your self-care strategies, such as vitamins and minerals, or herbal medicine. The combination of healing strategies will vary from woman to woman—one remedy doesn't suit all. Finding the right combination that works for you comes from your capacity to listen to your body, as well as getting good health information from qualified practitioners.

Initiating your healing journey

To ease you gently into the journey of healing your body, the following are two simple exercises you can do in the comfort of your own home. You'll discover they are surprisingly effective if you practise them over time. At the very least the exercises will help you to tune into yourself and create a greater feeling of calm and focus.

A simple yoga pose for easing cramps and PMS
Practised regularly Baddha Konasana, or Bound Angle Pose, is a safe way to soften and relax the abdomen, ease menstrual pain and heaviness, as well as help hormonal balance and premenstrual symptoms. Baddha Konasana promotes good blood flow throughout the pelvis, benefiting digestion as it frees the stomach and allows the colon to relax. This pose also assists gentle emotional release.

Baddha Konasana

To begin, sit on the floor with the soles of your feet together and your heels as close to the perineum (the area between your vagina and anus) as possible. Gently stretch your spine both into the ground, by pressing your sitting bones into the floor, and up into your neck and skull, tipping your chin slightly down towards your chest. Breathe naturally.

As you inhale, gently extend your spine, and as you exhale, gently lengthen your legs from your hips to your knees as you press your heels together. You will probably feel a stretch in your inner thigh muscles and your knees may naturally soften towards the floor.

You can practise a variation of this pose lying down, which is wonderful after coming home from work or at the end of the day. Begin as before with your soles together and heels close to the perineum. Lie straight back, with a small towel rolled as a neck rest if necessary, and with the backs of your hands on the floor, about 30 degrees out from your body.

You can also practise this posture with your feet slightly raised resting on a cushion or pillow—this is especially useful if you experience any backache when lying down in this pose. Raising your feet will relax and soften your pelvic cavity even further and can be very useful for alleviating menstrual pain.

To deepen your relaxation, throw a blanket over your body once you're in the posture and place an eye-bag or soft scarf over your eyes. Allow your eyes to sink deeply into their sockets. Relax and breathe freely.

You can stay in Baddha Konasana for up to twenty minutes—you may like to set a timer so you can relax more easily. To come up out of this pose, place your left hand underneath your left knee and manually lift it over to your right knee as you roll over to the right. Stay lying on your side for a couple of breaths and then gently come up onto your knees when you're ready.

If you like to multi-task you can easily practise this pose, the sitting version at least, while you're reading, watching television, meditating or just resting. Stay in the pose only as long as you're comfortable. To relieve menstrual and premenstrual symptoms you can slowly build up to five or ten minutes a day, two or three times a day throughout your cycle.

I did the pose with the soles of my feet together every day for a few months and was amazed—all my PMS symptoms went away and my period lightened and was pain free. To my surprise I really enjoy my periods now.
KARRIE-ANNE, 33

Psst . . . want to feel sexier and ease your period problems?
Known and practised for at least 4500 years in Taoist China, the Deer Exercise for women works through the endocrine system helping to naturally and gently balance your hormones and cycles. Women today have found it to be very helpful with premenstrual symptoms like bloating, feeling vague, fatigue, headaches and moodiness as well as irregularity, heavy bleeding, painful periods, lumpy breasts and polycystic ovarian syndrome. And, it can boost your sexual energy and improve your skin.

Eliza would bleed for anything between ten and twelve days, but after only two months of the Deer Exercise she reduced it to four to five days. Her moods are more even now and she's more patient and doesn't get nearly as drained. 'I have been in and out of hospital with my problems and had been told it was all psychological. I came to the Deer Exercise with no real expectations and have achieved far more than I ever planned,' she said. 'And as an added bonus, people have been commenting on how good I look . . . my skin has improved with all the broken capillaries gone.'

For one week every month Sally Anne didn't have a life, her PMS was so bad. Having discovered the Deer Exercise, everything has changed. 'Now I have no worries,' she declared.

My cycle has been regulated to 28 days on the dot, I don't experience the clumsiness, no longer endure sore, swollen breasts or fluid retention in my abdomen. I have even experienced totally symptom-free cycles and my period is now lasting only two to three days.

LEAH (AFTER DOING THE DEER EXERCISE FOR A FEW MONTHS), 39

The Deer Exercise

The Deer Exercise is very easy, takes little time and space and may be practised clothed or naked, seated on the floor or on a chair or the edge of a bed. Make sure you're warm and have privacy for about ten minutes. Start by sitting comfortably with your back reasonably straight, supported by the back of a chair if that helps. Close your eyes and focus on your breath, enjoying a few moments of peace and stillness.

To begin the exercise sit so that the heel of one foot presses against the mouth of your vagina and your clitoris. If this is too difficult you can position a tennis ball to create the pressure there.

Rub your hands together until your palms and fingers are hot—you may like to add a little oil to lubricate your hands if they're dry.

Place your hands over your breasts and, focusing on them, allow the heat to penetrate deeply. Gently begin to massage your breasts in a circular motion using the first three fingers of each hand and avoiding your nipples as these can easily be overstimulated. Continue this circular massage for a minimum of 36 rotations to a maximum of 360 rotations.

You can massage your breasts in either direction, outwardly or inwardly, depending on your own needs. Outward motion is called *dispersion* and is achieved by massaging along the underside of your breasts, your hands coming close together in the middle as they massage up towards the top of your breasts and out towards the edges along the top of your breasts and then down the outside edges of your breasts. Massaging in this direction may reduce the size of large breasts and reduce lumpiness.

Massage in an inward motion is called *stimulation*. To do this massage from the outside in along the top of the breasts, your hands come close together down the inside edge of the breasts and out from the centre to the edges along the underside of the breasts. This direction is not recommended if there is a history of breast cancer in your family—and massaging in this direction may increase the size of smaller breasts.

To absorb the energy you have generated through the massage to rebalance your endocrine system, place the tip of your tongue against the roof of your mouth just behind your front teeth—this helps connect the endocrine energy circuit within your body. Clench your anal and vaginal muscles as though you are drawing them up into your body and hold. As you do this maintain your awareness between your eyebrows. In this way the energy you have generated draws up through the endocrine system to the pineal gland, the uppermost endocrine gland. You can repeat the contractions three or four times, holding for 20 to 30 seconds at a time. Relax.

Within the first few times you practise the Deer Exercise you'll begin to feel the energy rising to your pineal gland. Maintain your focus on the area between your eyebrows. Many women find this is accompanied by feelings of peacefulness and expansiveness. Others see colours between their eyebrows. There's no right or wrong, just notice what *you* experience. If you have conditions like fibroids or ovarian cysts it may take you longer to feel the energy movement.

Many women have found that by persevering with the Deer Exercise and focusing their awareness keenly they can begin to shift stagnation in the body and experience this energetic movement. Similarly, as this energy moves it can gather in other parts of the body where healing is required; this may be felt like pins and needles or tingling or as if a cold area is gradually being warmed up.

You can practise the Deer Exercise once or twice a day, depending on the severity of your symptoms. You may like to start more intensely and then ease off to minimal or no practice as required. As a therapeutic practice in your self-help toolbox the Deer Exercise can be invaluable.[5]

CHAPTER 28

WHAT *YOU* CAN DO FOR YOUR PERIOD AND SKIN PROBLEMS

When I don't 'fight' my cycle and rest, pain and discomfort are greatly reduced and some months I feel a quiet joy in my femininity.

KELLY, 35

At 28 Annalise suddenly felt ready to take charge of her own health—to heal her endometriosis and PMS, which she had suffered from for some years. She had tried various therapies in the past and was ready now to focus on self-care strategies. 'This time the biggest difference is just a sense that my health is a real priority.' Having made a definite choice and knowing herself better, she's taking things slowly. As she says, 'Basically I have a playful approach to my choices.'

Having received menstrual health guidelines from her therapist Annalise stuck them on her study wall. She then has put gold stars by the practices she's been able to successfully do, such as less coffee and sugar, changing to non-toxic house cleaning and body products, eating lots of organic vegetables and fruit, having Epsom salts baths and resting when she bleeds. After only three months there's been quite a shift: 'I have much less PMT madness and pain. There's still that big pull inwards, and I feel tired, but the actual level of pain and irritability is something like 80 per cent less.'

It's empowering to be in charge of your own health—to feel you can make a difference. Naturally, where symptoms are extreme you'll also need ongoing and quite specific support from a holistic health practitioner. However, whether your symptoms are mild or severe, whether you see a health practitioner or not, it's what you do yourself on an ongoing basis that is the foundation for healing your period and skin problems.

In this chapter you'll find more specific information relevant to your particular condition that builds on what we've already outlined in the previous chapter. Check through the relevant parts and, like Annalise, pick those practices you feel you can comfortably start with. To shift more extreme conditions such as endometriosis or polycystic ovarian syndrome may require quite focused and intense treatment. If that feels overwhelming take your time to build up the healing practices. The most important thing is to keep going with them. And even if you do decide to go down the route of surgery for, say, your endometriosis or fibroids, remember that it's still vital to do the self-care practices to stop the condition from returning.

There are many vitamin, mineral and herbal supplements that can help enormously with period and skin problems. However, we generally recommend that you see a practitioner to get the best combination for your specific needs.

Often our long-term, deep healing comes through the very simple—more rest, more love, doing the work we love—going back to the basics.[1]

LARA OWEN, TEACHER AND AUTHOR

Premenstrual syndrome

Be prepared! *Always* know where you are in the cycle so that you're aware of when you're moving into 'that time of the month'. Being prepared also means under- rather than overbooking the diary, keeping your schedule as light as possible in this phase. And plan for some personal space where you don't have to take care of anyone else.

Eat magnificently—regular meals full of fresh vegetables, fruit, protein and whole grains. Avoid all soft drinks, sugar and sugar substitutes, refined carbohydrates, foods with synthetic additives and preservatives and all junk food. Carry wholesome snacks with you for the premenstrual blood sugar swings. Don't rush, skip or in any way compromise your meals leading into your period.

Minimise alcohol in general and avoid it in the days before bleeding. Make sure you're well hydrated by drinking plenty of water. This is very important if you suffer from headaches during your period.

Exercise is vital. As part of your program, do consider the yoga pose or the Deer Exercise that we described in the previous chapter. And also make sure to get plenty of natural light.

Tap into your period power. You may be having trouble getting real with yourself and others. Take some time to write in your journal about what's not working in your life, and who or what upsets you. Or perhaps you need to take more personal space, saying no to others more often. Value your feelings rather than dismissing them as 'that time of the month'. Protect your sensitivity by not pushing yourself—burn the 'to do' list—do nothing, simply rest.

I have found comfort and relief in understanding the pattern of my cycles, in understanding myself in those moods and moments where I might otherwise feel out of control.

MEGHAN, 22

When you're feeling good, write a letter to yourself about all your strengths: what you like and can celebrate. Read this letter when you're feeling down.

Unplug yourself—from technology, that is—as you come into your period and on that first day of bleeding. Plug in to you instead.

Practise stress reduction techniques such as the Emotional Freedom Technique or Thought Field Therapy. You'll find websites for further information on these in the Resources section at the end of the book. They are highly effective self-help processes for emotional and physical problems and are easy to learn. You can practise them on a regular basis as well as during menstruation.

If you're a smoker or take drugs, we urge you to quit now. There are many programs to help you to do this that include techniques such as hypnosis, Emotional Freedom Technique, neurolinguistic programming, acupuncture and the twelve-step programs.

Period pain

Follow the good food guidelines outlined in the previous chapter, avoiding junk and deep-fried and oily foods. But make sure to include the good oils—essential fatty acids such as flaxseed, evening primrose oil or fish oils. Increase your intake of foods rich in magnesium (like seaweed, almonds, dates, rice, cashews, walnuts, brazil nuts and spinach) and calcium (like sesame seeds and tahini, almonds, seaweed, dark green vegetables and sunflower seeds). Always make sure the nuts and seeds are raw and as fresh as possible. If they taste rancid throw them out.

Just before and during bleeding eat small, easily digestible meals. Avoid constipation by drinking plenty of water, eating a fibre-rich diet and avoiding wheat and soy products. Soaked prunes and apricots, and calcium-rich foods may help but make sure you get Vitamin D— remember, it's free from natural light—to metabolise the calcium. Although it tastes a bit unpleasant a small amount of raw potato juice can

Drop your bundle!
Rest, go slowly, work
your schedule to
accommodate the
symptoms, and move
at the pace that your
body would like to
move at and not your
brain. This eases
tension, which in
turn will ease your
symptoms.

also work wonders, as well as slippery elm powder mixed with a little freshly squeezed orange juice. And if none of this works seek support from a holistic health practitioner, and in particular check for candida and allergies.

Read Chapters 20 to 26 on period power and notice what most catches your attention—that could be a key to your healing.

Consider doing the Deer Exercise daily and the yoga pose described in the previous chapter, as well as learning some other yoga poses. Avoid wearing tampons and luxuriate in an Epsom salts bath or two.

I had horrific pain at the start of my period for about the first two days, and this had been the case for about ten years, and it became progressively worse. After using ONLY cloth menstrual pads for nine months I was completely free of that 'uterus twisting' pain that I thought I had to live with. No more tampons for me!
MARIAM, 35

Endometriosis

As endometriosis is quite a severe condition you'll need to follow the health rules for period pain as closely as possible. Make a healthy diet your priority and especially address any digestive problems such as allergies or candida.

Find ways to reduce stress overall in your life. Use the cycle as your guide, as described in the chapters on period power. Make the days of your period or the ones that are most painful as restful as possible. Always wear pads rather than tampons, and even consider cloth menstrual pads—they're so gentle on the body and there are some pretty gorgeous designs available which make having periods feel more special. Learn meditation or the Emotional Freedom Technique mentioned in the PMS section.

Take more time to deeply rest at your period.

Reduce your toxic load by using only the safest cleaning and body products. Avoid all synthetic perfumes, incense and candles. Consider purchasing an air purifier or ioniser especially if you live and work in the city. Develop a varied, sustainable exercise program. It might include a gentle-ish workout at the gym, walking, Pilates, tai chi or yoga. You'll also benefit enormously from working closely with a holistic health practitioner such as a Traditional Chinese Medicine or Ayurvedic practitioner, a naturopath or homoeopath.

Amelie had a very positive story to tell. While in labour with her first child, the doctor on duty asked about the scars on her belly. She informed him they were from surgery for her endometriosis. 'So, this is an IVF baby', he replied. Amelie was able to proudly announce that, no, it wasn't an IVF baby, but naturally conceived and surprisingly quickly. Endometriosis can cause infertility, although it wasn't the surgery that made the difference to her symptoms. Rather, she saw a chiropractor who used kinesiology, and an acupuncturist, and combined this with her self-care practices. After only about three months she had, in her words, 'spectacular success' in reducing her symptoms. Although she waited two to three years before she tried to conceive, she went on to have two healthy children both conceived and born naturally.

Irregular cycle

Start charting the cycle you do have, including observations of the physical changes, such as mucus and temperature. Check the Resources section for where you can learn fertility awareness methods. You can always start with the Menstrual Dreaming Chart described in Chapter 20: 'What's the point of a cycle?' The act of charting will help you to be more aware of your body and feelings. Awareness alone can start to shift things and help you to get in touch with period power.

If your life is all over the place aim to find ways to bring more rhythm or regularity to it in general, like having a more regular sleep pattern and eating regular meals—based on the good food guidelines, of course. Have some protein at every meal and in particular include a small portion of full fat organic yoghurt in your diet daily. Research has shown a link between low-fat dairy in the diet and increased risk of infertility due to lack of egg release—also known as 'anovulatory infertility'.[2] Enjoy being in nature and getting as much natural light as possible.

If you're someone who's pretty driven and doesn't get much downtime, then you'll need to address that. Also, overexercising can stop your period and weaken your bones. Make sure you get sufficient rest and recovery time while enjoying a sustainable and varied exercise program. Try the Deer Exercise as a low-impact practice that is great for balancing your hormones, and will leave you feeling calm and nourished. Therapies such as acupuncture can be very helpful.

Polycystic ovarian syndrome (PCOS)

Follow the guidelines for irregular cycles. It's vital that you eat a really nourishing diet that includes lots of mineral-rich green leafy vegetables. Avoid refined carbohydrates, sugar and low-fat foods. Eat some protein at every meal, and try replacing grains with beans and lentils. Make sure to get essential fatty acids such as flaxseed oil, evening primrose oil or fish oils.

Exercise is important, especially if you're overweight. The good news is that you only need a 5 per cent drop in weight to regulate your hormones. The importance is regularity of exercise, not intensity. Try walking for half an hour daily.

Dr Christiane Northrup recommends that you look at any negative childhood messages you may have taken on about being a fertile woman. Bring these internal messages to consciousness so that they don't control your body or your ovaries.[3] Enjoy discovering your period power.

As this can be quite a difficult condition to heal we encourage you to work closely with a holistic health practitioner.

Dealing with my PCOS has taught me a lot about the power of the body-mind connection. I'm learning to say 'Yes to Mess!'—more willing to have my life changed in pace and rhythm by my cycle, more accepting of my vulnerable, erratic feelings premenstrually and the sheer messiness of the blood. Making this inner shift along with changes in diet, using acupuncture and Chinese herbs makes me feel I am healing my body and deepening my sense of who I am as a woman.

SARAH, 35

Fibroids

Clean up your diet by removing all junk food. Drink plenty of water and lemon water (see previous chapter for the recipe). You could benefit from a strenuous exercise program, as well as practices such as the Deer Exercise.

Above all it's very important to reduce your environmental load, similar to endometriosis sufferers, including stopping the use of tampons. Fibroids will naturally diminish with falling levels of oestrogen as a woman goes through menopause.

You would also benefit from seeing a naturopath or other holistic practitioner. Research has shown some success with Traditional Chinese Medicine.[4]

Heavy bleeding

Clean up your diet and your environment. Take more time to deeply rest at your period. The Deer Exercise is excellent for reducing excessive bleeding so it's well worth making this practice a priority.

You may find it a good idea to give up tampons. And, strangely, quite a few women have commented that they bleed less when they wear *cloth* menstrual pads. The duration of Nina's period went from five to six days down to about two days. Then, when she didn't use the cloth pads, her period took about four days.[5] Try them—they're soft and comfortable and, like Nina, you might just bleed less.

Skin problems

Good skin comes from the inside out, not the outside in.[6]
MARK HYMAN, MD

Eat a great diet that includes lots of fresh vegetables and fruit and in particular avoid highly processed and fatty foods—that is, deep-fried and oily food, soft drinks and refined sugar in general. Include the good oils that we've mentioned in the PMS section. Go easy on alcohol and make sure you are well hydrated by drinking plenty of water. Eat only whole fat dairy such as organic yoghurt. Retrospective evaluation of the Nurses Health Study found that women who frequently consumed low-fat dairy such as reduced-fat milk, skimmed milk and cottage cheese as teenagers were more likely to suffer from severe, doctor-diagnosed acne at the time.[7]

An antibacterial face wash can stop pimples from getting infected—a few drops of tea tree oil in warm water is all you need. Try a face pack made from yoghurt, honey, lemon, orange juice (you can add a little olive oil if you have dry skin) and kelp powder to draw out the impurities.[8]

People have been commenting on how good I look . . . my skin has improved with all the broken capillaries gone.

ELIZA (AFTER DOING THE DEER EXERCISE FOR A FEW MONTHS)

Get some natural light each day for at least ten minutes—before 9 am in the southern hemisphere and between 8 am and 8 pm during daylight hours in the northern hemisphere. Consider vitamin and mineral supplements and herbal remedies prescribed by a naturopath. Supplements such as Vitamins A, E and B6 have proved helpful.[9]

Check for food allergies. In one study almonds, malt, cheese, mustard, red pepper and wheat flour (in that order) caused the greatest exacerbations of acne. Milk may also worsen acne too.[10] Acne can be due to candida overgrowth and toxin accumulation in the gut—seek professional support to deal with this and to balance your hormones.

Exercise, as ever, is great. And, finally, do be patient with the healing process; this one may take a little time.

CHAPTER 29

HOW YOUR CYCLE IS CONNECTED TO YOUR RELATIONSHIP

The menstrual cycle can support you in building a healthy relationship but when it's not understood or appreciated it can sometimes feel like a troublesome, disturbing force!

John was a bit confused with his partner Fran's mood swings because there was no explanation. 'As a man I have no natural cycle, no way of counting the days and weeks, no knowledge of what it's like to have a cycle. I found it hard to equate depression with a physical process. I don't understand why you'd let it happen,' he says. But because Fran is now very open about her PMS, it's easier to cope with, and he can understand it more.

Many men can find the cycle a real mystery but respond well to information and, when they do understand, can be very supportive of their partners and benefit themselves from knowing about period power. And some men find women who enjoy their natural cycle just plain sexy.

Luke is one such man. He has an almost visceral reaction against the Pill. He's always been into a healthy lifestyle and wouldn't want a woman to compromise herself in that way. He instinctively senses that such a compromise would affect him too. 'I just can't imagine doing it to myself, so I wouldn't expect it from them. I just enjoy women . . . I think men are fairly ignorant of the menstrual cycle, it's that time of the month when they can't rationalise with their partner and it's just better to go surfing!' But he's found that he can experience more intimacy with women when they bleed because of their greater sensitivity and softness.

> The cycle can provide rhythm for a relationship—the times when you're out there doing lots of things, the need to be chilled and quiet together, the need for time apart, a time for sex, a time for emotional connection that's not sexually charged, and the need for the occasional good healthy fight!

The menstrual cycle can help to build healthy relationships

William, a man in his mid twenties, thought he'd done something wrong in the first few months of his relationship. He could feel a change of mood in his partner, Cassie, in the getting real phase that made him feel uncomfortable. She'd say it wasn't him, and so he learnt to just 'be' there, let her be and not take offence. At her period she's more inward. Now when she needs space, he's happy to back off, and when she needs him to be there, he's happy to do that when he's able to. He sees no reason to create tension, treating her changes as normal and healthy. He enjoys supporting her in the rhythm of her cycle because it benefits him, too. Instead of going for a run, they'll be more quiet and reflective, perhaps going for a gentle walk together instead.

Cassie loves how William is extra thoughtful about her at her period. Without being asked he'll offer her a massage. Learning to negotiate the cycle has created more intimacy and tenderness—they enjoy good communication, and that's probably the secret ingredient that allows things to flow well between them.

Along with providing a rhythm for your own life, the menstrual cycle can also provide a rhythm for your relationship. There'll be times when you want lots of connection and times when you need to be getting on with your own thing; times of strong sexual desire and times of none, times when you love every millimetre of your partner and times when you wonder what you are doing with this person. All normal.

You may notice that these different experiences of your partner might have a pattern that's in sync with the different phases of your cycle. Once your period is over and you're moving towards ovulation, connection with your partner may tend to be easier, and as you draw towards bleeding it may become more challenging or provocative.

At ovulation I feel sexy and glowing and want to get close to my man.
ANYA, 28

The 'getting real' days leading into the period can include having a bit of an emotional purge. If this phase is a hotspot in your relationship, it may be an indication you're both avoiding dealing with issues. Like a lightning conductor, a woman can sometimes become the channel for picking up the unexpressed charge or repressed stuff in a relationship.

Libby has a habit of dumping boyfriends the day before her period. It's like a wild force that rips through her, always the day before bleeding. If she's not tracking her cycle it can catch her unawares. It's as though she's overwhelmed by all the things that aren't working for her and getting out seems like the only solution. Remembering that this is 'the great reality check moment', Libby has to decide how much her reaction is a failure to address issues throughout the month, for which her partner must also take some responsibility, and how much it's her deep inner wisdom telling her that this relationship really isn't for her. Either way it does require some serious inner reflection and a difficult conversation or two with her partner—both of which are worth doing.

A man would be wise to pay attention at these times rather than dismiss it as 'that time of the month', because he can get useful feedback on how the relationship is travelling as well as an opportunity to learn things about himself and his partner.

The process of charting my cycle affected the quality of my relationship; the awareness of the cycle, the conscious choices for contraception and conception, became an intrinsic part of the rhythm of our sexuality and a rich and juicy part of the relationship.

ELLA, 35

Men and PMS

Some men can be acutely aware of their partner's cycle if she suffers badly from PMS, alerting her when her period might be due, or taking precautionary measures to minimise any upset. While it's great that a man can be tuned in to that extent, in anticipating the arrival of the period, there's a danger that he may end up 'walking on eggshells' around you, trying to 'be good' so as not to exacerbate the situation and, therefore, not caring for his own needs sufficiently.

Paradoxically, such behaviour can sometimes end up bringing on the very thing he wanted to avoid. You may feel humoured or patronised and this can also be bad news. He may not fully understand why you're reacting—after all, he's being 'so reasonable'—but underneath there's an implied message that something is wrong with you. At this point, a man may be starting to feel as though he can't win. He's his usual self and he cops flak, and he tries to do the right thing and cops flak again.

There are no innocent parties. Recent research has found that PMS is worse for women who are in a relationship with a man than for those who are in a same-sex relationship. This suggests that men can be a catalyst for or contribute to PMS. Yep, that's right, men can cause PMS.[1]

Professor Jane Ussher found that when women were asked to give an account of their PMS, many spoke of a relationship issue. A woman would attribute a problem to PMS when often it was a quite reasonable issue to be upset, angry or frustrated about in her relationship with her partner. In current research she's exploring how much a partner's reaction to premenstrual stress impacts on the woman and the degree to which relationship issues actually cause or worsen a woman's premenstrual distress. Ussher says men need to be better equipped to respond to a partner's symptoms, and appreciate the role they can play in magnifying or mitigating the pain.[2]

It was a couple of days before my period and my head was saying 'Don't speak, don't speak' but the words flew out anyway! They were quite harsh and critical. Normally I'd suppress such thoughts but I couldn't . . . actually it turned out to be really positive. After the initial reaction we had a marvellous, honest discussion that really shifted things in our relationship. And I ended up feeling proud of that 'difficult' voice in me.

ALI, 42

In the 'getting real' phase you may be unable to hold back your feelings. You may be less tolerant, or some things he does may irritate you. You may be more assertive in relation to your own needs and less sensitive to him. Or, maybe you just want more support. Some of this may cause discomfort in your partner but that doesn't mean you're doing anything wrong. It's important that you're taken seriously and that the issues you raise are addressed. When a man ducks and weaves around an issue it only adds to the tension.

Having said that, he doesn't have to accept behaviour that's hurtful or abusive. A woman needs to learn how to communicate her needs without attacking or 'losing it', and equally men need to appreciate how they can contribute to an outburst by their failure to take responsibility for some aspect of the relationship. Your partner may not always be able to do what you ask but simply engaging with the issue is important. If your partner is emotionally dependent on you, he might suffer when you need more time for yourself. You may find his needs 'too much' and may indeed get frustrated and reactive. You want him to take responsibility for his own feelings and not depend on you so much.

The more you let your partner know about your needs and feelings at different times of the month, and the more both of you take the time to really listen to each other and respect each other's needs, the less reactive both of you will be. The mirroring exercise described in Chapter 31: 'Negotiating contraception' is an invaluable tool for helping you deal with this.

Interestingly, if a man finds a woman's 'getting real' phase difficult because she seems reactive, he might want to consider that some women on the Pill can be permanently tetchy and reactive. One young man, who was well versed in the dangers of the Pill, would bet his friends in high school that he could tell which of the young women were on it. His clues were pasty skin, rather 'tight' body movements and an irritable, touchy disposition. He was usually right.

Men change too

The myth is that men don't change—they do. Men are no less subject to cycles than women, the obvious ones being the day–night and seasonal rhythms. Some men may even be sensitive to the changing phases of the moon.

Monica noticed that coming into the dark of the moon each month, Richard would go into a distinctive downward spiral, losing hope and feeling lots of self-doubt. She'd immediately think, 'where's the moon?' and invariably it was entering the dark phase. She shared her observations with him, although it took him about six to eight months to fully 'get it'.

> Research that took out any reference to the menstrual cycle found that women and men equally have fluctuations in energy and mood.

Now he's proactive, using it as his 'getting real' time. With this awareness he feels more in control, and the downtime is less of a drama. And as he says, 'I'm also having a feeling of belonging and not feeling so separate, it's pretty special.' He's getting a great insight into how the menstrual cycle might feel for women.

If men can appreciate how their own emotional life can fluctuate, they may be more accepting of our rhythmical patterns. Their feelings may not surface so readily the way ours do, or even follow a pattern like the menstrual or lunar cycle, however, men are equally full of feeling. They may not outwardly appear cranky, irritable or vulnerable, but being silent and unresponsive could be a result of those feelings *in* them. A man may simply deal with it in a different way. Vulnerability, or the need to withdraw, might see him zoning out in front of the telly or playing a computer game for hours on end.

Interestingly, research that took out any reference to the menstrual cycle found that women and men equally have fluctuations in energy and mood. It explored changes through the week with depression and anxiety peaking on Tuesdays and good cheer peaking on Fridays. These mood cycles were observed in women and men. And, as Karen Houpert pointed out in her book *The Curse*, while these ups and downs were found to be greater than those reported with the menstrual cycle, there's been little time, energy or money spent to find 'a cure' for these distressing weekly mood swings.[3]

> [T]he human body is like a river constantly in the process of change ... your body is not the same at seven o'clock in the morning as it is at seven o'clock in the evening.[4]
>
> **DEEPAK CHOPRA**

Deepening emotional intimacy

Instead of regarding the 'getting real' phase of the cycle as a problem, you can both use it constructively to do a bit of emotional and relationship 'house cleaning'—all relationships thrive on regular check-in times even if the conversations get a bit tense. Such clearing prepares you both for the highly sensitive and charged state of menstruation when you can potentially open to a more blissful connection. Naturally, opening to the bliss does require some emotional effort and care, and you may not have the luxury of time and space for that every month. However, the more you can access that heightened place with ease, the more your partner can join you there.

While you can't mechanically program for this bliss spot, there are certain things both of you can do to allow for it. Be in tune with the cycle and know roughly when your period is due. Slow down both your schedules in preparation for it. Create some quiet time together, respecting the high sensitivity of this time. It's *because* of this sensitivity, and your ability to come into the relationship with it, that allows you both to experience greater levels of connection.

This space is highly charged and the vulnerability of intimacy is sometimes 'too much'. Because of this we can easily flip into the opposite, clashing and detaching. It was the day before her period and Anna thought she was doing really well having avoided any tension, but her partner gave her 'a look' over something that at any other time she might have ignored, but on this occasion it got to her and they ended up arguing.

> It's because of this sensitivity (at menstruation), and your ability to come into the relationship with it, that allows you both to experience greater levels of connection.

Billi discovered this special intimate space by chance while away on a romantic weekend with her lover, and they were both

> Think of yourself as holding the key to a sacred intimacy that your partner can be drawn into if he's ready.

already in a very relaxed space. She happened to bleed. She remembers that night before the blood actually started flowing as one of her most exquisite, loving experiences. They didn't have wild sex, but found themselves lying together for hours in a deep state of connection.

Now is the time as the woman to drop your agendas on what you 'ought' to be doing and simply let things be. And be immensely tender and kind with yourself. Think of yourself as holding the key to a sacred intimacy that your partner can be drawn into if he's ready. The man needs to drop out of 'doing' mode and pay attention to the clues from his partner, and ask her what she wants. Some women prefer intimacy without sexual pressure at this point in the cycle. Generally she doesn't want any demands made of her, she simply wants to 'be'. Join her there—hang out, be close, listen, respond and be gentle. It's this delicacy that can open the door to deeper union (and could lead to wonderful sex). And some women have a powerful surge of sexual energy during their period that is anything but tender. What can we say . . . enjoy!

> *I love having a partner who's open to living with and supporting a natural woman and being part of my sexual and fertility cycles and aware of sharing natural contraception responsibilities.*
>
> **GAYLE, 37**

Loving the cycle

If men are to relish a woman's menstrual rhythm, then above all we women must make peace with it. The challenge for women is to accept that it's OK to change: that you can be easygoing and tolerant one minute and then demanding and assertive another; that you can feel full of energy, drive and a desire to socialise and at another time want to chill out. There's nothing 'wrong' or selfish about standing up for yourself or needing to be on your own. It's all part of healthy self-care.

Men also need to remember that the qualities most associated with menstruation—high sensitivity, deep feeling, intuition, dreaminess, the need to be alone, ecstasy and passion—are the ones that our culture least values.

The cycle can provide rhythm for a relationship—the times when you're out there doing lots of things, the need to be chilled and quiet together, the need for time apart, a time for sex, a time for emotional connection that's not sexually charged, and the need for the occasional good healthy fight!

A man can be a great ally for a woman when he openly respects her cycle—enjoying her changing rhythms, affirming her singular power and depth at her period, and being able to join her in that heightened place of bleeding. You as the woman can give him the key as a man to enter a gorgeous place of ease, intimacy and sexual union that will cast a glow over your whole relationship life. The more men understand period power, the more illogical the Pill will seem to them and the more they will want to do their bit for contraception.

CHAPTER 30

THE SLOW ROUTE TO A GREAT RELATIONSHIP

Clarissa and George dived into the deep end of sexual intimacy the night after they first met, enjoying the intensity of their instant romance. Living in different cities acted as a speed bump, so to speak, slowing down the pace a little, but still, after two months—out of nowhere, it seemed to Clarissa—George suddenly announced that he felt overwhelmed by the speed and intensity of the relationship. Initially they weathered this disturbance, but the relationship has now ended with some considerable distress for Clarissa.

There are important ingredients for creating a long-lasting relationship. Some are obvious, like good communication, respect for your partner, respect for yourself and being able to experience sexual pleasure together. But in our fast-paced lifestyle one vital ingredient we often overlook is the importance of taking time. Clarissa and George tried the fast route to sexual and emotional intimacy and came unstuck.

In the past I've gone straight to sex as a way to get close to someone but in retrospect that didn't serve me. I know what I was after but it didn't work.

ELOISE, 35

To get more from life and to feel more alive we spoke, in Chapter 21, of the Slow Movement that celebrates such things as slow food and slow cities. To that list we now add slow relationships. Remember that 'slow' refers not only to taking more time to do things, but also to allowing everything its own timing, and not imposing an artificial pace. We might have speed dating, but speed doesn't work if we want to form a long-term relationship. It often happens that after going full on into a relationship, one or other of the partners suddenly gets overwhelmed, announcing, rather like George, 'I need space, this is going too fast for me'.

Of course, there's nothing wrong with wanting to have sex straight away when the attraction is strong. Many of us have been there. However, there's also real pleasure in getting to know someone the 'slow way'. And there's less chance of being left so vulnerable and confused if it doesn't work out.

Relationships have their own magical timing and part of the adventure and richness of relationship life comes from being able to honour that timing instead of trying to hurry the journey to intimacy. In this way you engage with the philosophy of 'slow' and can start to enjoy getting to know someone at a more measured pace, rather than leaping straight into the deep end of sex. In this way you can build true intimacy.

Kate has had a couple of relationships and enjoyed her fair share of one-night stands but at 21 feels ready for that long-term relationship. 'One-night stands don't sit well with me now,' she said. Interestingly, she's also found she can't experience orgasm if she's not friends with the guy. With friendship she feels respected and that allows her to relax. Now she wants to wait for a relationship to emerge and allow time to work its magic before having sex again.

I went on the Pill for three days once. I didn't like the effect on my body
or my mind. So, was I now meant to casually sleep with anyone
I fancied? I realised that wasn't really how I liked to operate . . .
So I stopped taking it.

MICHAELA, 42

Going on a journey

Beginning a relationship is like embarking on a journey with gorgeous, wonderful sexual and emotional union as your destination. Getting to know each other, getting to know yourself more, and how to be together with each other's quirks and complications are some of the steps along the way. How well you handle these challenges will give you clues about whether the relationship is going to last or not, as well as building your emotional intelligence skills.

Emotional intelligence means that you're more in touch with your feelings, are able to soothe yourself when you're distressed, can trust your feelings to give you guidance on what is good and not good for you, and also how to communicate them in a way that they can be received by others. All this takes time but is essential for creating a great, long-term relationship and taking sex to deeper levels of connection.

Building a relationship slowly is like savouring each mouthful of a beautiful meal, rather than gulping it down. When you eat fast you miss all the delicate and complex flavours and dull your tastebuds.

On the surface, I know as a man I have benefited greatly from the Pill,
yet somehow, I feel a loss because of it. I'm not entirely sure what
this loss is, suffice to say, it's something I feel at a spiritual or
primordial level.

RUSSELL, 45

Relishing the slow gear

Intimacy thrives in 'slow' conditions. You can't *make* it happen, but the more you open to each other—let go, be vulnerable, patient and willing to have those 'difficult' conversations, the more you can grow into intimacy.

The Pill, by removing some of the natural checks and balances that slow down the journey to sexual intimacy, can artificially speed up a relationship. This has meant women can be sexually available at all times. However, being permanently available doesn't automatically equate to having satisfying sex or enhancing a relationship, even without the fear of getting pregnant. The very act of negotiating contraception is one of the stages of the relationship journey. It might be awkward, embarrassing, even challenging, but how you come through it will give you real clues as to whether the relationship is worth pursuing.

Amy was put on the Pill at the age of fifteen for period problems. Once she became interested in boys, she found being on the Pill 'took away my ability to say no'. It was as though she had no excuse anymore. Being a teenager with all its attendant insecurities, this is understandable. However, many women express the same difficulty, finding themselves saying yes to sex when, in hindsight, they'd have preferred to say no.

I felt bad about saying no when 'it's OK, you won't get pregnant'. I may not have had so many sexual partners either if I'd had more knowledge about my body.
ROCHELLE, 37

Interestingly, Peter, who instinctively feels the Pill isn't right and has seen girlfriends suffer with too many health problems, felt sexually pressured when a girlfriend was going on the Pill just for him. There was an expectation that they must now have sex, and it took away, for him, a more organic sense of timing about when it might happen.

If a woman is already on the Pill when she comes into a new relationship, she may not know what her 'timing' is. Fran was on the Pill for her PMS when she first met her husband, John. Initially it felt quite 'grown up' and sexually liberating to be 'in control' of her fertility. 'It was new and exciting to be this "mature" woman. I could offer myself to my new partner without bothering him with the "hassle" of condoms.' Fran might happily have continued using the Pill if it had eased her PMS symptoms, but it didn't. After three years, and after discussions with John, who was entirely supportive, she came off it when she found more natural ways of healing and valuing her cyclical nature.

Initially they used condoms, but are now practising natural fertility methods. Although John felt they had lost the spontaneity of their sex life, Fran is more relaxed and confident and now finds sex is 'very real, very connected and I can share my PMS matter of factly—it's just a diary date. He's now realising the complexity of me. Coming off the Pill I've had to learn to communicate intimate things. I grew up not talking about this even with myself.' John and Fran are now more present with each other and their sexual expression has been enriched.

I learned that in order to get closer to my lover I had to get closer to myself first.[1]
DIANA RICHARDSON, AUTHOR AND TEACHER OF TANTRIC SEX

The rhythm of sexuality

Your sexual drive isn't a static, 'same all the time' experience. It changes as you change, waxing and waning with the rhythms of your menstrual cycle.

Our sexuality has many moods or gears, from deep and dark to light and playful and everything in between: loving, passionate, flirtatious, provocative, exquisite, tender, forceful and much more. The trouble with taking the Pill is that it knocks out many of the sexual nuances and, in effect, flattens your sexual life.

The Pill seems to neutralise women. There's something mysterious and dangerous about the menstrual cycle.

DAVID, 49

Andrew finds that sex can be more intimate and relaxed when his partner is on the Pill, because she's not anxious about getting pregnant. This is understandable. However, it's also a compromise. You might be able to enjoy sex on the Pill but, if you want to experience deeper emotional and sexual intimacy, the Pill will often block this. A woman on the Pill can be shut off from her emotional depths. As a man you want her depths as much as your own to keep growing into a greater union.

When she has her period Cassie feels that 'it's my time, my body's time' and she doesn't want sexual contact. But after the period she's more sexually charged because she's held back. Laila, on the other hand, feels an enormous sexual drive during menstruation—hungry and wild and quite different from her experience of the sexually high time at ovulation, which she feels is more about pleasing her partner.

Are you ready for the next level of sexual experience?

There's the C-spot (your clitoris), the G-spot (inside the vagina on the front wall, about 2.5–5 centimetres in size), the A-spot (a patch of sensitive tissue at the uppermost end of the vagina near the cervix), the P-spot (the perineum—the area between the vagina and the anus that's full of sensitive nerve endings) and the U-spot (a small patch of sensitive skin on either side of the urethral opening) as well as *so* many different sexual positions you can explore to make sex exciting. Were you also aware there's a whole other level of sexual experience that you can enjoy beyond spots and techniques? And you guessed it, it's another of those slow movements. Commonly known as Tantric sex this approach has also been called slow sex.

Now I really love myself and my orgasms are beyond anything I ever dreamed.
ANNETTE, 42

Just as we encourage you to be aware of and feel into the different energies and moods of your cycle and the power of simply letting go at menstruation to get that delicious natural high, so the instructions are similar for Tantric sex. In Tantric sex the emphasis is on slowing down and become more present to yourself—your internal movements of energy—rather than focusing on outer expression and technique. It requires letting go, presence and vulnerability and that opens you to an exquisite sensitivity, revealing 'a magnetic layer of excitation in the body that is cool, cellular and ecstatic'.[2]

Tantric sex is about slowing it down and being present to all the sensations and all life and making sexuality sacred.
CATHY, 29

In her book *Tantric Orgasm for Women*, Diana Richardson describes two types of orgasm—peak and valley: 'peak orgasm depends on an active build-up of excitement and the valley orgasm arises from relaxation'.[3] Our usual mode of sex is focused on getting peak orgasms, while the Tantric sex approach introduces us to valley orgasms. It's as though in truly letting go you can release the orgasmic potential of the *whole* body.

There's no sudden change or technique involved but rather a shift in consciousness that evolves through stillness, observation of all the subtle changes and refinement of your experience. As you do this you may feel 'a coming home', as Annette did when she discovered Tantric sex five years ago. 'It was easy,' she said. 'I didn't have to try so hard, I could just be who I am. As I relaxed I became aware of the sexual energy that was already there in my body, and it really started to flow.' It was the art of *feeling* rather than *thinking about what she was feeling* that made all the difference. Annette had struggled for years with her body image, and had even been bulimic. The process of Tantric sex has allowed her to let go of that, and as she says, 'It certainly makes sex a lot better now that I'm not thinking about how big my bum is! Now I really love myself and my orgasms are beyond anything I ever dreamed.'

Cathy has always looked for depth in relationships and exploring Tantric sex has allowed her to find that depth. 'It's been incredibly satisfying,' she said.

When a woman learns how to nourish a romance with her own body to unite with it from the inside, alive in all her senses, she exudes a breathtaking feminine quality that transforms the atmosphere around her.[4]

DIANA RICHARDSON

The Pill has made men lazy lovers

While Diane Riley, co-author of *Sexual Secrets for Men*, is grateful for the liberation that the Pill gave women, she's conscious that it's put women's sexuality on tap for guys and that there's more pressure on women to be sexually ready when emotionally they're not. 'It's penis-focused sex, penis in vagina: him and her come. They lose out on exploring all the other pleasure zones of the body. Men are rewarded for being lazy lovers.' And ironically both parties can end up feeling empty and unsatisfied.

Petrea and her boyfriend have just begun exploring Tantric sex. While her boyfriend was happy to go to a workshop together, she's noticed that if she doesn't bring it up they slip back into their usual sexual practices, which are OK, but she now knows there's more than that. She also wants off the Pill. She sees the Tantric approach as offering them more creative ways of enjoying sex without the risk of pregnancy during her fertile times, but initially it would demand more of her boyfriend. 'Life's pretty easy for him right now,' she says, 'but it could get a whole lot better for both of us if we were a bit more adventurous.'

On the other hand Meghan and her partner were already an experimental couple sexually and being off the Pill actually played to their strengths. As she said, 'The Pill doesn't challenge you to be creative with intimacy and with love. Suddenly we were forced to be more creative . . . and it was beautiful.'

Tantric sex offers you more options for experiencing sexual pleasure without the risk of getting pregnant. However, the important thing to remember overall is that there's no right or wrong way to approach sex. It's about making choices for what you want to enjoy while being mindful of contraceptive needs.

There's a huge and rich body of knowledge to discover in Tantric sex and we encourage you to check out some of the literature. Our favourites are books by Diana Richardson and Margo Anand. And there are also some websites for more information in the Resources section of this book.

> *The Pill doesn't challenge you to be creative with intimacy and with love.*
> *Suddenly we were forced to be more creative . . . and it was beautiful.*
> **MEGHAN, 24**

The convenience myth

The Pill is touted as a great convenience for women. You take it once a day and then don't have to think about contraception any further. Or, if you have an implant or an injection, there's even less to worry about. However, convenience doesn't create a healthy relationship or great sex. In the same way that we're now waking up to the problems of convenience or fast foods, we need to start questioning the convenience of the Pill.

We've alluded to the high cost of not valuing Nature's cyclical life in farming practices. For women who are taking the Pill, a similar cost is being accrued: a cost to your health and fertility as well as to your emotional life and relationships—none of which is 'convenient'. The pressure of speed and the shallowness of convenience can leave us feeling empty and disconnected. Separation and divorce rates may be as high as they are in part because we have lost the slow cooking time that is required for a relationship of longevity and depth.

CHAPTER 31

NEGOTIATING CONTRACEPTION

You've decided to come off the Pill but your partner isn't keen on using condoms. Or perhaps you've just started going out with someone, the attraction is building and pretty soon you're going to have to discuss contraception.

Sex *is* exciting stuff, with the potential and promise of deeply pleasurable energy exchange, loving intimacy and sharing and acceptance of your innermost self. Discussing contraception may not be the most exciting part of your sexual relationship, nevertheless the quality of this dialogue and shared responsibility can add enormously to the trust, relaxation and intimacy of a sexual relationship—all factors that can enrich your sexual experience.

I wouldn't have asked a man to take the Pill and yet I took it myself unquestioningly.
It was my boyfriend who was concerned that the Pill wasn't good for my health.
Together we explored other means of contraception.
BILLI, 38

Like any other major relationship decision, what to do about contraception needs careful thought and discussion. First, you'll need accurate information about a variety of methods. Secondly, you'll need to hear each other's concerns, worries and preferences. And, thirdly, you'll need to *spend the time it takes* to come to a contraception plan that really works for both of you. This is an ongoing process—as your relationship evolves, as issues of fertility and sexuality unfold, as you gain more understanding of contraceptive methods and options, and as your circumstances change. The time taken to attend respectfully and consciously to the issue of contraception, even if this involves a swathe of messy feelings, is invaluable in nurturing your relationship.

Generally speaking, sharing responsibility hasn't been our recent cultural expectation of contraception in committed relationships. Past the 'protection against sexually transmitted disease' stage, contraception has largely come to be seen as the responsibility of women. This imbalance in responsibility and decision-making often leads to resentment, which in turn insidiously, and sometimes terminally, undermines a relationship.

My boyfriend of six and a half years became very complacent. He refused to change to condoms so I could have a break from the Pill and I felt like he took my sexuality for granted, which I resented. Now I'm off the Pill it's made such a difference to how my current partner perceives my sexuality. It's great to share the contraceptive responsibilities.

MELINDA, 33

Jacinta really suffered on the Pill, with bouts of depression, weight gain, lethargy and feeling 'just not right'. She was overjoyed to learn about fertility awareness. Throwing away her pills, she excitedly began charting her cycle but the reception from her boyfriend was considerably less enthusiastic. 'He sat there looking stone-faced and upset. I don't remember him saying too much, but it really hurt me that he couldn't seem to understand my excitement or enthusiasm.'

Change can be difficult at the best of times, so it's very important that both parties engage in the conversation from the beginning, however self-evident the outcome may be for the woman. Sadly, Jacinta's relationship didn't last. Perhaps it might have helped if she'd shared more of her distress about the Pill and her discovery of fertility awareness. It would have allowed her boyfriend more time to adjust to the idea and learn about other options for sexual pleasure without the risk of pregnancy. Alternatively this change may have revealed the fault lines in their relationship and simply hastened its ending.

Exploring options

Through the life of a relationship a number of methods of contraception may be used. The more information about, and experience with, different forms of contraception you have, the more you'll be able to choose appropriately, lovingly and safely at different times and under different circumstances.

In addition, experimenting with forms of lovemaking that don't lead to a risk of pregnancy can add deliciously to your options. Some couples decide to practise periodic abstinence at fertile times. Far from being a trial, many of those who choose this approach report that it enhances their sexual connection and love.

Other couples find their own way of managing their fertility. Lisa had been charting her cycle for some time before meeting her husband. As she was confident in her capacity to know her fertile and infertile times, her husband trusted the method and they settled into a lifestyle of sexual activity to fit in with where she was in her cycle: 'we have intercourse when I'm infertile and oral sex during my fertile phase—it's a great arrangement and we're both very happy with it'.

At first Samuel was very skeptical about fertility awareness, but once he understood it, he was truly excited and interested. Eventually, he was defending fertility awareness with his mother, who was worried that it was the rhythm method!

MEGHAN, 22

Communication for greater intimacy

If approaching the subject of contraception is difficult and you feel communication between yourself and your partner could do with some improvement, you're not alone! Communication—real, honest and respectful—is perhaps the primary and perpetual work of relationships. If you put in the time and effort to learn and practise good communication skills, it will strengthen and enrich your relationship, and quickly erode it if you don't. It takes two! There are many useful books and courses available, and it's well worth gaining some expertise in this area. You may also surprise yourself with how much more there is to know about each other and how fun and moving these processes can be.

The following process, 'mirroring', is one such exercise and has been adapted from Harville Hendrix's book *Gettting the Love You Want*. It's very helpful for practising respectful communication between partners, in which each of you can feel really *heard* and your various feelings, opinions and concerns respectfully *included*. Mirroring is also known as reflective, or active, listening.

Mirroring

In this exercise you'll learn to send clear and simple messages, to listen carefully to what your partner has to say, and to paraphrase your partner accurately. This will lead to clear and effective communication. Allow yourselves 45 minutes to an hour.

Choose one of you as the initial 'sender'. This person says a simple statement that begins with 'I' and describes a thought or feeling. For example, 'I woke up this morning and felt anxious about going to work'. At the practice stage it's recommended that you choose fairly neutral, but real, statements. Starting with a highly charged

---

issue will tend to undermine the exercise as emotions may be too intense for partners to pay attention to learning this new skill.

If the sentence seems too complex, the receiver can ask for simplification: 'Could you say that in fewer words?' Once a clear and simple sentence has been sent, the receiver paraphrases the message and asks for clarification. For example: 'This morning you woke up feeling that you'd rather stay home than go to work. Did I understand what you said and felt?' Asking for clarification is important, as it shows a willingness to try to understand.

The sender responds by saying, 'Yes, you did', or by making a clarifying statement, such as: 'Not exactly. I woke up this morning wanting to go to work but worried about what was going to happen.' This process continues until the sender is able to say that what was said had been accurately heard. Then, the sender and receiver switch roles and communicate another simple statement, processing it in the same way as before.

Practise this technique several times until you become familiar with the procedure.[1] Initially it may feel like an unnatural, awkward way of relating, however, it's an invaluable way to learn accurate communication, and the skills, once learnt, do become natural and automatic. You can then start to use your new skill communicating about issues that may be more charged. Remember to take turns. When it's your turn to listen, give your partner your full attention. Ask clarifying questions, but don't try to analyse or interpret. When, and only when, you both feel heard and understood you can begin to find solutions that will work for you both. You may want to do this later, allowing time for all that you have both heard and said to 'compost'. The expanded options arising out of this sort of process will enhance your relationship and are just plain sexy. You'll see!

For Meghan and Samuel going off the Pill was a decision they negotiated together, although it took some time for them both to be comfortable about it. They went for private sessions with a fertility awareness trainer. 'At first Samuel was very skeptical,' Meghan said, 'but once he understood it he found it truly exciting and interesting. Eventually, he was defending fertility awareness with *his* mother, who was worried that it was the rhythm method!'

Now that they're practising fertility awareness, both Meghan and Samuel need to be conscious of the sexually charged time around Meghan's ovulation. Meghan has found, 'There is something very primal and feverish and beautiful going on inside me, and those root energies are very difficult to say "No" to!' Because of this they've realised the importance of taking responsibility together and their sex life now feels 'incredibly fulfilling'.

After talking to my partner we came to a decision where we both had to be responsible for contraception and we feel fine about it. I actually feel more like a true woman as I have to look after my own fertility . . . Our sex life is better like this. We both have become more conscious of natural cycles.

BONNIE, 31

What to do in brief encounters

In brief sexual encounters, where practising communication skills and relationship building may not be top of your list but contraception and prevention of sexually transmitted diseases are, the means for these still need to be negotiated. This will usually be brief as well, and even non-verbal, but it certainly helps to be aware of what your own requirements are before going ahead.

Clearly in brief encounters condoms are essential to prevent sexually transmitted diseases being passed between yourself and your temporary partner. Condoms, used correctly, are also reasonably effective contraception, however, as you're unlikely to want to get pregnant you may wish to back this up with a diaphragm or spermicide or by knowing whether or not you're fertile.

Taking the Pill as backup for brief encounters means permanently being subjected to all its effects for what are, perhaps, sporadic sexual encounters. You may feel this is overkill and too high a price to pay since there are alternatives that will work just as well when you need them and enable you to hum along to your own natural rhythm in between times.

Discussing contraceptive failure

Sex is powerful in its capacity to create human life and many of us are testimony to the fact that even when contraception was used, the potency of our parents' fertility was the greater force.

The common misunderstanding that the Pill is *almost* 100 per cent effective and therefore the only real contraceptive option has meant many couples fail to anticipate the possibility of an unplanned pregnancy. The truth, of course, is that any form of contraception can let you down and this can be very stressful, especially if you and your partner have never discussed it and suddenly find that you have different views as to what you want to do about the pregnancy and your relationship. As always, prior discussion can be helpful, before things become so critical and imminent. Along with your careful consideration of contraceptive options, it's wise to discuss your thoughts and feelings about an unplanned pregnancy, before the fact if possible, while being aware that you may feel differently when, or if, an unexpected conception occurs.

> Taking the Pill as backup for brief encounters means permanently being subjected to all its effects for what are, perhaps, sporadic sexual encounters.

What about children?

Have you had a chat with your partner about children? Do you want them? Does your partner? Will they have red hair and green eyes? Be Catholic or pagan? A team, or just one each? This can be fun, scary, gruelling or just where you're heading next. Many couples avoid this discussion, assuming the other wants what they want, only to be disappointed and hurt when this proves not to be the case.

With the advent of the Pill and the *concept*, at least, of totally reliable contraception, as well as relatively safe abortion and sterilisation, we're now in an age that offers men and women sexual relationships *and* the choice as to whether they want children or not. Children by choice are by definition wanted children and research has shown that wanted children tend to be better cared for and become more caring and contributing adults. However, while this choice can certainly be empowering it may be difficult for some to consciously choose parenthood or find the 'right time'.

Furthermore, either or both of you may have mixed feelings about your fertility or ability to get pregnant. Even if you're not really planning children just yet, you may be thinking, 'I wonder if I can get pregnant?' 'Wouldn't it be amazing to have a baby together?' 'What would our kids look like?' 'Am I shooting blanks?' After all, sex and love do tend to bring up cluckiness and family kinds of thoughts, even though you may be making a conscious daytime decision that now is *not* the time for a baby.

To manage this conflicting mix, it's good practice to recommit to your contraceptive choices—each cycle at your period is an obvious time. In this way you can be completely clear that you don't want to get pregnant during *this* cycle, while not discounting future possibilities.

The couples known to be the most casual about their contraception are those who have a child, or children, and are planning more. Very often their attitude is, 'We're not trying just now but it's OK if it happens'. If this is you, it's still worthwhile making a month-by-month decision so that you can consciously plan an optimum pregnancy. Then again, some people just like a surprise!

EPILOGUE: CONTRACEPTION FOR GREAT SEX

How can we celebrate and enjoy our glorious sexuality without dreading getting pregnant and without damaging our bodies or cutting off whole swathes of our emotional, sensual and creative life?

Books on relationships and sexuality generally don't discuss contraception. And yet what you choose for contraception and *how* you go about choosing it can enhance or diminish your relationship and sexual connection. If you make these choices haphazardly or unconsciously—by following the crowd or based on insufficient advice—then this can lead to resentment and distance in your relationship rather than sexual intimacy.

On the other hand, seeking thorough information about contraception, and making choices in a loving and supportive atmosphere, will most certainly contribute to the intimacy and trust in your relationship—important ingredients for great sex.

Genevieve tried a number of different methods of contraception, including the Pill and an IUD, then she learnt the Natural Fertility Management methods and found that this was just right for her. 'I *love* being in touch with my own rhythms and cycles, and knowing where I'm at fertility-wise,' she enthuses. Her partner Paul thinks, 'it's great living with a natural woman and being part of her sexual and fertility cycles'. Genevieve and Paul happily share their contraceptive responsibilities and enjoy using fertility awareness to decide about when, or if, they want to have children.

In the same way that relationships and sexuality are journeys of discovery, learning about your fertility and cycles can equally be an adventure that reveals new horizons.

Sex is a potent, grown-up activity, with powerful grown-up consequences—emotionally, physically, socially and psychologically. In order to experience all that sex offers—the fun and the passion as well as the fulfilment and healing—requires embracing the whole sexual package. By giving care to your decisions about contraception, as well as all the other implications of a sexual relationship, you may be very pleasantly surprised about what experiences unfold for you.

APPENDIX 1
HOW THE PILL DOES WHAT

As mentioned in the Introduction, we are, in writing this book, taking the liberty of considering all hormonal methods of contraception collectively—some of which are clearly not a pill—for the convenience of being able to discuss that which is the same, or similar, about these methods. Here, however, we'll separate them out, as the delivery and action of different methods of hormonal contraception vary, and we imagine you'd like to know *specifically* the action of the form that you are using, or are considering, or once used.

Brand names of formulations will vary from country to country, and even within a particular country the same formulation may be produced by different drug companies and have different names (and different prices). More to confuse us!

The International Planned Parenthood Foundation has a very comprehensive website with a directory listing all forms of the Pill and other hormonal contraception throughout the world, the regional equivalents of different brand names and their component hormones and doses. If this sounds useful go to www.ippf.org and check it out. You'll need to register, but it's free.

Combined oral contraception

There are basically two types of Pill currently available. The most commonly used are combined oral contraceptives (COCs), which contain synthetic oestrogen and progesterone. These have either the same oestrogen and progesterone dose throughout the cycle, or have variable quantities of these hormones creating two or three phases during the cycle.

The hormone levels in COCs are similar to a state of early pregnancy: by making your body think it's already pregnant, COCs stop your ovaries from producing eggs—a sterilising effect—and your uterus from developing an egg-receptive lining—an abortive effect. It also makes the mucus in your cervix thicker and much more difficult for sperm to swim through and into the uterus and Fallopian tubes in their search for an ovum to fertilise. This is a contraceptive effect.

COCs are taken as a daily dose, most often with 21 days of hormone pills followed by seven days of placebo pills, allowing for a withdrawal bleed. The withdrawal bleed experienced by women on the Pill is often mistakenly called a 'period' but is simply a result of stopping the drug. This is not the same as a natural period that occurs following ovulation during your normal menstrual cycle. The 21:7 ratio of hormone to placebo pills characterises COCs currently available in Australia.

Other COC formulations vary: for example, Seasonale™, available in the United States, has 84 days of hormonal pills followed by seven placebos, and Minesse™, available in Europe, has 24 days of hormonal pills followed by four placebos.[1 & 2] Newly released Anya™, in the United States and Canada, and Lybrel™, in Britain, have been designed to be taken 365 days a year.

Progesterone-only pills

We also have progesterone-only pills (POPs), often called the mini-Pill. By containing no oestrogen, progesterone-only pills don't inhibit ovulation, but work primarily by thickening cervical mucus and, secondarily, by preventing the uterus from preparing its egg-friendly lining: effectively, contraception and abortion. Some POPs contain higher doses of synthetic progesterone, which will also inhibit ovulation in most cycles, adding sterilisation to the way this form of contraception works. It has not been approved for use in all countries, where the Pill (in the form of COCs) is otherwise available.[3 & 4]

Injectables and implants

Injectables and implants are ways of delivering synthetic hormones without having to remember daily pill-taking.

Depot medroxyprogesterone acetate (DMPA) is a progesterone injected directly into the muscle of your upper arm or buttock every twelve weeks. Its most common brand name is Depo-Provera™, but there are others. As a higher dose of progesterone than the POPs, DMPA works by preventing ovulation and the lining of the uterus from developing as well as thickening cervical mucus.

Implants are also a progesterone-only form of contraception. They are generally a little smaller than a matchstick (a 40 millimetre by 2 millimetre ethylene vinyl acetate rod) and are inserted directly under the skin of the inside upper arm by specially trained doctors. They work via continuously releasing the synthetic progesterone etonogestrel into your bloodstream over three years. After three years the implants become less effective and need to be removed, also by a trained doctor. Approximately one-third of women who have implants have them removed less than twelve months after insertion.

Norplant™ was an early, and now discredited, implant and consisted of six rods. Currently the most widely known and used implant is Implanon™, which is a single rod, but there are others, like Norplant II™ and Jardelle™, with varying numbers of rods.[5 & 6]

Intrauterine devices

A recent incarnation of the earlier intrauterine devices (IUDs) is the levonorgestrel IUD (LNG-IUD) or intrauterine system (IUS), which is a small, flexible device made of metal and/or plastic inserted into the uterus, where it slowly releases the progesterone levonorgestrel over a five-year period. The progesterone content of these devices works similarly to other progesterone based contraceptives, thickening cervical mucus and making the uterine lining hostile to implantation. In some women ovulation is also prevented or delayed. A widely available LNG-IUD is Mirena™.

All intrauterine devices need to be inserted and removed by a specially trained doctor.

Other IUDs available release copper rather than hormones, and work by inhibiting sperm movement towards the uterus and Fallopian tubes, ovum movement down the Fallopian tube, fertilisation of the egg by the sperm, and implantation of a fertilised egg into the uterine lining.[7 & 8]

Vaginal ring

One of the more recently developed forms of hormonal contraception is the vaginal ring. It's a 54-millimetre ethylene vinyl acetate copolymer ring which a woman inserts into her vagina where it releases synthetic oestrogen and progesterone. The vaginal ring is another way of delivering the same hormones that are in the COC pill and has the same contraceptive effect.

The ring is inserted on day one, that is the first day of bleeding, of the cycle and is left there for three weeks before being removed for seven days, which allows for a withdrawal bleed. A new ring is then inserted. During the three weeks in which the ring is in place it may be removed for up to three hours without loss of contraceptive cover.[9 & 10] Nuva Ring™ is the most widely available brand of vaginal ring.

Transdermal patch

The contraceptive patch delivers synthetic oestrogen and progesterone through the skin via a 20-millimetre band-aid-like square stuck onto the skin of the buttock, upper outer arm, belly or upper torso (but not the breasts). A new patch is applied weekly for three weeks before a patch-free week allows for a withdrawal bleed. A new patch is applied after seven patch-free days.

Patches are yet another way of delivering the same hormones as the COC pill and, for contraceptive purposes, they work in the same way.[11 & 12] Ortho Evra™ is a common brand of contraceptive patch.

Emergency contraception

Emergency contraception in the form of a dose of synthetic hormones, commonly called the morning-after pill, is an abortifacient and not really a method of contraception at all. It's used as a backup method to prevent the implantation of a possibly fertilised egg at a time when no contraception was used or, if it was, its use was faulty (for instance, when a condom breaks).

In many countries, including Australia, the morning-after pill is available over the counter and elsewhere a doctor's prescription is required. It needs to be taken during the 72 hours after unprotected sex, although it's most effective in the first 24 hours. After 72 hours the morning-after pill can still be effective but its efficacy starts to diminish.

Several varieties of morning-after pill are currently used, although none is universally available. Mifepristone (RU486™) is one, Levonorgestrel (a progesterone) is another and the Yuzpe method another. The latter is a way of using whatever COC (for instance Microgynon-30™) is available—four tablets are taken: two to start with then another two twelve hours later. Nausea is a common side-effect of the morning-after pill and anti-nausea medication is often given at the same time. If the nausea causes vomiting, the effectiveness of the morning-after pill may be compromised.[13 & 14]

Convenient as the morning-after pill may be as a backup, we also need to be aware that these may have lasting side-effects as well. A British medical database has shown evidence that two or more exposures to levonorgestrel used for emergency contraception may triple a woman's risk of developing multiple sclerosis. And studies have found multiple use of the morning-after pill is linked to an increased risk of breast cancer.[15]

APPENDIX 2
THE PILL DISTURBS NUTRITION

Studies have shown the metabolism of these nutrients is disturbed when a woman uses hormonal contraception:

Vitamin A (retinol)
Some studies show an increase, and some show a marked decrease of beta-carotene levels in the blood. Beta-carotene is the Vitamin A precursor. This may lead to eye problems, susceptibility to infection, dry and scaly skin, lack of appetite and vigour, defective teeth and gums, heavy menstrual bleeding, cervical problems. Vitamin A is an important antioxidant and anti-cancer vitamin.[1]

Vitamin B1 (thiamine)
Studies show a likelihood of deficiency in Pill takers, which can lead to fatigue, weakness, insomnia, vague aches and pains, weight loss, depression, irritability, lack of initiative, constipation, oversensitivity to noise, loss of appetite or sugar cravings and circulatory problems.[2]

Vitamin B2 (riboflavin)
Taking the Pill leads to a deficiency of Vitamin B2, which can cause gum and mouth infections, dizziness, depression, eye irritation, skin problems and dandruff.[3]

Vitamin B6 (pyridoxin)
Studies show marginal to severe deficiency in Pill users, causing nausea, low stress tolerance, lethargy, anxiety, depression, weakness, nervousness, emotional flare-ups, fatigue, insomnia, mild paranoia, skin eruptions, loss

of muscular control, eye problems, herpes and oedema, impaired libido, impaired blood clot prevention.[4]

Vitamin B9 (folic acid)

Levels of Vitamin B9 are considerably reduced in Pill users, risking abnormal synthesis of DNA and congenital abnormalities including neural tube defects, spina bifida, deformed limbs and Down syndrome in a baby if conception occurs while on the Pill or in the period immediately after stopping. A deficiency may also lead to damage to the small intestine wall, anaemia and raised homocysteine levels, which are associated with cardiovascular disease, as well as various gynaecological problems and repeated miscarriage.[5]

Biotin

Levels of biotin are lower in women on the Pill. This nutrient helps to prevent the overgrowth of candida in the digestive tract. An overgrowth of candida is much more than vaginal thrush and leads to a whole raft of unpleasant symptoms, including sugar cravings, overall itchiness, allergies and asthma, chronic fatigue, anxiety, headaches and much more.

Vitamin B12 (cobalamin)

Levels of Vitamin B12 are reduced in Pill users, especially vegetarians, causing anaemia, a sore tongue, weight loss, depression and raised homocysteine levels (see Vitamin B9 above).

Vitamin C (ascorbic acid)

Pill use increases the breakdown of Vitamin C by up to 30 per cent causing bruising, bleeding gums, 'spider' veins, heavy menstrual bleeding, eye problems, loss of appetite, muscular weakness, anaemia, fatigue and lowered immune response. A deficiency will make it harder for the body to produce sex hormones when a woman comes off the Pill. The effectiveness of supplementation may be also reduced and taking Vitamin C while on the Pill can increase the concentration of oestrogen in the body, effectively turning a low-dose Pill into a high-dose one and increasing potential side-effects.[6] At the same time a high dose of Vitamin C (over 2 grams a day) can interfere with the effectiveness of the Pill.

Bioflavonoids (rutin, hespiridin, etc.)
Body levels of bioflavonoids are decreased during Pill use. These essential nutrients are part of the Vitamin C complex and have an effect on capillary strength and blood pressure. They also contain anti-inflammatory properties.

Vitamin E (mixed tocopherols or alpha tocopherol)
Women on the Pill have an increased need for Vitamin E as it is used to normalise the higher oestrogen levels in women on the Pill—except for those taking the mini-Pill. Blood plasma levels of Vitamin E are *lowered* by about 20 per cent with Pill use. This deficiency causes anaemia, muscle degeneration, subsequent low fertility, changes in the menstrual cycle and hot flushes. Vitamin E is also needed to offset blood clot formation and the possible carcinogenic effects of oestrogen.

Vitamin K (menadione)
Pill use leads to higher levels of Vitamin K which in turn may lead to blood clot formation.

Iron
Less iron may be lost menstrually for those women for whom the Pill causes lighter periods. This may alleviate anaemia for those women who suffer from iron deficiency.

Calcium
Absorption is greater on the Pill—another plus!—however, as critical ratios of calcium to other minerals are disturbed, this can lead to a whole raft of health problems.

Magnesium and potassium

Although there is no conclusive study that we know of linking lowered magnesium and potassium levels with Pill use, clinical evidence indicates that deficiencies of these minerals are very common in women on the Pill. This can cause premenstrual symptoms, lumpy breasts, muscle cramps, anxiety, sleeplessness, chocolate or sugar cravings and cardiovascular problems. After ceasing the Pill production of fertile mucus may be affected until normal levels return.[7]

Selenium

Levels of this antioxidant are reduced by Pill use. Selenium has been shown to reduce the chances of deformity, including Down syndrome, in children. This protective effect is lost in pregnancies commenced while on the Pill or soon after stopping.[8]

Copper

Absorption of copper is increased in women on the Pill, raising the need for Vitamin C and disrupting the zinc/copper balance. This can lead to immune dysfunction, insomnia, mental turmoil, mood swings, irritability, depression, migraine, hair loss, high blood pressure and clotting tendencies. This has serious implications for many aspects of pregnancy and foetal health. In extreme cases low zinc and high copper is implicated in schizophrenia.[9]

Zinc

Zinc levels are significantly reduced in Pill users, which can lead to diabetes, sugar cravings, loss of appetite, poor resistance to infection, skin infections, lowered fertility, impaired normal growth, cell division and tissue repair. Zinc is crucial for many processes during pregnancy and needs to be adequate before conception. Long-term Pill users may find it difficult to raise their zinc status to adequate levels.

Prostaglandins

Levels of certain prostaglandins are reduced with Pill use. Prostaglandins are normally made from essential fatty acids and use zinc as a catalyst. They're intricately involved in hormone production, relative levels of pain experienced and blood clot formation.

Blood lipids

Low and very low density lipids, cholesterol and triglycerides, are increased in women on the Pill, raising the chances of heart disease.

Serum proteins

The levels of serum proteins, or proteins in the blood, are all altered by Pill use.

APPENDIX 3
WHAT ABOUT A PILL FOR MEN?

Since the first Pill was released in 1960 we have frequently heard about research into a contraceptive pill for men, and sometimes about its imminent approval and release. Nearly fifty years later this still hasn't happened, and we may wonder: is it likely to?

After grave problems with the earlier oestrogen-only Pill, in the 1970s Doctors John Rock and Gregory Pincus tried out the first combined synthetic oestrogen and progesterone Pills on a Harvard volunteer group and some chronically ill mental patients. Both men and women took a high-dose form of Enovid (10 milligrams) that was more than enough to stop ovulation in women and sperm production in men. One of the men displayed shrunken testicles and all further trials by these researchers on a male Pill were abandoned. They agreed that any male Pill would have to be *really safe* before experiments could proceed.[1]

From time to time various other attempts have been made to find a male hormonal contraceptive but none has become available—either the side-effects have been deemed unacceptable or the drug or method unmarketable.

Current research that 'looks promising' and may produce results within the next few years is based on a long-acting testosterone ester coupled with synthetic progesterone delivered by injection or implant. The progesterone suppresses spermatogenesis (creation of sperm) by acting on the pituitary, similar to the suppression of ovulation by the Pill in women, while the androgen (male hormone) content maintains 'masculinity' and libido. Concerns exist about the very careful balance needed between efficacy and the risk of the drug promoting aggression, enlarged prostate and the susceptibility to arterial disease.[2]

We wonder if it is indeed possible to strike such a universal balance considering the differences in physiology and biochemistry of individual men, and the variations within an individual man over time. From our experience of women and the Pill we may be right in thinking it's not possible to interfere with a man's profoundly sensitive hormonal make-up without side-effects.

While not a pill the intra vas device or IVD system is another method of male contraception that is still being researched. You'll find details of this method in Chapter 16.

Men and women are different

Let's consider here a fundamental difference between men and women in terms of health management. For a long time now many of the female reproductive processes have been medicalised and pathologised. Menstruation, childbirth, breastfeeding, menopause—as well as female organs themselves—and have become the province of medical intervention in epidemic, and often unnecessary, proportions. Think: high caesarean section and hysterectomy rates, elective plastic surgery, breast implants, hormone replacement therapy as well as the therapeutic and contraceptive use of the Pill. While we can certainly be grateful for life-saving drugs and procedures, it seems we're not striking a balance between these and what we can best manage naturally for ourselves.

By and large we women are not encouraged to positively engage with our bodies and their changing processes. Much as we may joke about male egos and men's relationship with their penis, we may also notice that men often have more respect for the integrity of their bodies. At the risk of stating the obvious, a fundamental physiological difference between men and women is that it's women who get pregnant and bear children. In all likelihood this means women have a greater contraceptive motivation and *willingness* to do harm to themselves in order to prevent an unwanted pregnancy.

Whatever the cause of our different relationships with our bodies, perhaps we women can take a leaf from the blokes' book of physical integrity. Instead of wishing for a male contraceptive pill that may interfere with *their* health and wellbeing, we can start to practise a healthy suspicion about any drug or device that interferes with *our* natural feminine processes.

APPENDIX 4
ENVIRONMENTAL SIDE-EFFECTS

There are many chemicals that find their way into the environment that are known to affect our endocrine system, which in turn can affect our hormonal balance. These include pesticides, surfactants for removing oil, chemicals used in some commercial spermicides, some dental sealants, certain chemicals used to seal canned foods, and others used to soften materials made of plastic, like 'rubber' gloves, intravenous bags and baby bottle nipples.

Similarly, the active oestrogenic ingredient of the Pill—not including the mini-Pill—has been identified as a potential endocrine disrupter.[1] Other forms of hormonal contraception with an oestrogenic component are the emergency contraceptive pill, the contraceptive patch and the contraceptive ring.[2]

The Pill is intentionally designed to disrupt the natural functioning of a woman's endocrine system. However, it also acts as an endocrine disrupter when released into the natural environment via sewage. These chemicals have been shown to then affect both fish and human beings.[3]

Lifelong exposure to such oestrogenic endocrine disruption in some fish populations has been found to cause *complete reproductive failure* within one generation.[4] The British Environmental Agency examined ten lowland rivers over a five-year period. As a result of oestrogen in urine from the Pill passing through sewerage works they found 50 per cent of male fish had developed eggs in their testes and in many cases had developed female reproductive ducts.[5] Behavioural effects have also been noted; for instance, female mice exposed before and after birth exhibited masculinised behaviour as adults.[6]

There is also evidence to suggest that exposure to environmental oestrogens may be having adverse health effects on humans.[7] These include the dramatic decline in sperm count and quality, an increase in the incidence of some reproductive cancers like breast and prostate, premature puberty, and increased incidence of endometriosis.[8]

One of the main issues guiding recent research is the relative environmental impact of some of the newer hormonal contraceptives. The contraceptive patch and contraceptive ring could pose even more ecological risks after disposal than oestrogens in urine. A used patch flushed down the toilet or sent to a landfill can harm wildlife as it continues to release the hormone ethinylestrodiol.

Swedish scientist Joakim Larsson estimated that relatively few patches flushed down the toilet could have a negative impact on the environment. It was calculated that a single patch flushed every three days would shed enough hormone to impair fish—that is, damage their ability to reproduce—downstream from a particular Swedish sewage treatment plant.[9] While the manufacturers of the patches agreed to warn Europeans not to flush or incinerate the products, no such warning exists in Australia or the US. Even if warnings are given it would be impossible to police their disposal.

A used contraceptive ring, like the Nuva Ring™, has similar environ- mental effects. Upon disposal, a contraceptive ring has a third more oestrogen than a month's worth of discarded patches, or six times more than a month's supply of birth control Pills.[10] It's estimated that a used contraceptive ring still contains approximately 2.4 milligrams of ethinylestrodiol. This is enough to taint 24 million litres of water to a concentration that is biologically active in fish. Instructions are included with rings telling users not to flush them but, as with patches, this doesn't ensure compliance. A ring can also be accidentally expelled while a woman is on the toilet.[11]

Clearly hormonal contraceptives can have side-effects that range far beyond those experienced by an individual woman.

APPENDIX 5
MY CONTRACEPTION PLAN

To clarify where you are at contraceptively, and how you may improve your protection and experience, fill in the blanks and cross out those words that don't apply to you.

Date:

I/we need contraception every day/ every week/ sometimes/ occasionally/ not at all. I/we also need/don't need protection from sexually transmitted diseases (STDs).

I/we currently use _____ for contraception/STD protection.

One being totally unhappy and five being totally happy, I am/we are one/two/three/four/five about the contraception/STD protection I/we use.

For backup contraception/STD protection I/we use _____. I/we could also use _____.

One being totally unhappy and five being totally happy, I am/we are one/two/three/four/five about the backup contraception/STD protection I/we use.

I/we would like to find out more about _____ as possible method/s I/we might like to use.

I/we would like to try/to learn about _____ to use for contraception.

Steps I/we can take to improve my/our contraceptive experience, under-standing and cover: _____

_____

_____

_____

_____

We recommend you make copies of this blank plan and use them to review your contraceptive plan every six months to one year until you're completely happy with your use and understanding of your chosen method(s) of contraception. Then, review at times of change, like after a baby, after a period of celibacy or at the beginning of a new relationship.

APPENDIX 6
MY MENSTRUAL DREAMING CHART

On the first day of your period you can start recording your thoughts and feelings on day one of the Menstrual Dreaming Chart. Watch the pattern of your cycles unfold as you continue to record over a number of months. Begin a new chart at the start of each period.

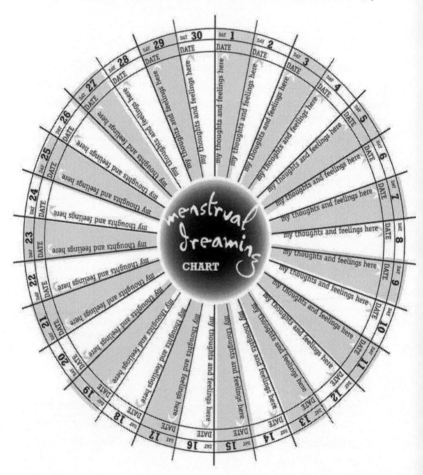

RECOMMENDED READING AND RESOURCES

For information on the Pill and other forms of chemical contraception

John Guillebaud, *Contraception: Your Questions Answered*, Churchill Livingstone, Edinburgh, 2004.

Christine Read et al., *Contraception: An Australian Clinical Practice Handbook*, Sexual Health & Family Planning Australia, Ashfield, NSW, 2006.

Sherrill Sellman, *Mothers Prevent Your Daughters from Getting Breast Cancer*, GetWell International, Tulsa, OK, USA, 2003.

World Health Organization, Medical Eligibility Criteria for Contraceptive Use and *The Selected Practice Recommendations for Contraceptive Use.* These publications are available online at: <www.who.int/reproductive-health/publications/mec/andspr/>.

The International Planned Parenthood Foundation has a directory of comprehensive hormonal contraceptives. You will need to register to use this directory, but it's free: <www.ippf.org>.

For information about the pharmaceutical industry

Lynne McTaggart, *What Doctors Don't Tell You*, Thorsons, London, 1996.

Ray Moynihan and Alan Cassels, *Selling Sickness—How Drug Companies Are Turning Us All into Patients*, Allen & Unwin, Sydney, 2005.

No Free Lunch: a coalition of doctors opposed to the overt and covert inducements offered by the pharmaceutical industry to 'encourage' doctors to prescribe their wares. They believe a doctor's first responsibility is to the patient, not to the shareholders of drug companies: <www.nofreelunch.org>.

For fertility awareness information, counselling and resources

Francesca Naish, *Natural Fertility*, 4th edition, Sally Milner Publishing, Bowral, NSW, 2004.

Francesca Naish and Jane Bennett, *The Natural Fertility Management Contraception Kit*, NFM Kits, Sydney, 2004.

The Jocelyn Centre for Natural Fertility Management and Holistic Health is a specialist naturopathic fertility clinic in Sydney which offers natural contraception and programs for pre-conception health care and treatments for fertility problems. You can also enquire about Natural Fertility Management (NFM) trained counsellors in your area as well as how to become an NFM counsellor yourself. Francesca's books and the NFM kits are available from the clinic and website. Francesca Naish is the founder and director and the contact details are, phone: +61 2 9369 2047 and website: <www.fertility.com.au>.

Also check out <www.nfmcontraception.com> which has loads of information about the Natural Fertility Management methods, articles and a free calculation service if you had a surprise conception you believe may have been the result of spontaneous ovulation. You can also purchase an NFM contraception kit from this site.

Natural Fertility and Women's Health offers specialist naturopathic fertility treatment in New Zealand. You can contact Jo Barnett for an appointment, a referral to a practitioner in your area or an NFM Contraception Kit, phone: +64 3 960 4926 and website <www.natural fertility-womenshealth.co.nz>.

Justisse Healthworks for Women offers fertility awareness education, holistic reproductive health care, holistic reproductive health practitioner training, and therapeutic counselling. Geraldine Matus is the founder and director of The Justisse Method and is based in Edmonton in Canada. The contact details are, phone: 780 420 0877 or 1-866-JUSTISSE (1 866 587 8477), and website: <www.justisse.ca>.

The Fertility Awareness Center provides instruction in secular, sympto-thermal fertility awareness. The Fertility Awareness Network is a coalition of teachers of fertility awareness, primarily in North America, but also other English-speaking countries. Ilene Richman is the director and the contact details are, phone: 212 475 4490 and website: <www.fertaware.com>.

Taking Charge of Your Fertility is a website offering fertility awareness software, charts and discussions focused on fertility, health and family, and is based on the book *Taking Charge of Your Fertility* by Toni Weschler. Website: <www.tcoyf.com>, and in Australia and New Zealand <www.lullabyconceptions.com>.

The Garden of Fertility is a website offering fertility charts, amazing photographs of the cervix during the menstrual cycle (including a woman on the Pill), discussions and articles, books and a study guide if you want to teach fertility awareness. Website: <www.garden offertility.com>.

The Billings Ovulation Method websites have extensive information about this method and results from worldwide trials. Websites: <www.billings-ovulation-method.org.au> and <www.woomb.org>.

For good reading about relationships and sexuality

Margot Anand, *The Art of Sexual Ecstasy: The Power of Sacred Sexuality for Western Lovers*, GP Putnam & Sons, New York. Margot's website: <www.margotanand.com>.

Mantak Chia, *Taoist Secrets of Love: Cultivating Male Sexual Energy*, Healing Tao Books, Huntington, New York, date unknown. This book has information on how to achieve male orgasm without ejaculation.

Thomas Moore, *The Soul of Sex*, HarperCollins Publishers, New York, 1998.

Diana Richardson, *Tantric Orgasm for Women*, Destiny Books, Rochester, 2004. Diana's website: <www.livinglove.com>.

You can also check out these websites:

<www.oztantra.com.au>.

<www.australianschooloftantra.com.au>.

<www.bluetruth.com>.

<www.relationships.com.au> The website of Relationships Australia.

For good reading, and watching, about women's power and the menstrual cycle

Jean Shinoda Bolen, *Urgent Message from Mother*, Conari Press, York Beach, ME, 2005.

Giovanna Chesler, *Period: The End of Menstruation*, <www.periodthemovie. com>; an hour-long documentary about menstrual suppression.

Alexandra Pope, *The Wild Genie: The Healing Power of Menstruation*, Sally Milner Publishing, Bowral, NSW, 2001.

Alexandra Pope, *The Woman's Quest—Unfolding Women's Path of Power and Wisdom*. A thirteen-session self-guiding course, self-published in 2006. Available from <www.wildgenie.com>. Alexandra's website also explores women's ways of accessing power and knowledge, understanding the wisdom of our cyclical nature and creating menstrual wellbeing, as well as information about her workshops, counselling and coaching.

Other interesting websites:

<www.shetime.net> encourages women to see their natural monthly cycle positively, to respond to it creatively and to share their experiences and tips.

<www.menstruation.com.au> has lots of information and products, and offers an alternative and very positive viewpoint about menstruation.

<www.moondiary.com.au> You can order a moon diary and other 'tools for the journey' featuring lunar lore, moon stories of many cultures, and ideas for simple but powerful rituals.

<www.redwebfoundation.org> The site of The Red Web Foundation which promotes menstrual health through community and education.

<www.yoni.com> Discussion, celebration and products of all that is woman. Check out the gorgeous yoni, or vulva, puppets available from this site.

<www.recreatingmenstruation.com> Information and women's discussion of the Deer Exercise. You can also purchase Lisa Bodley's ebook on the Deer Exercise.

<www.menstruationresearch.org> The site of the Society for Menstrual Cycle Research—a scientific organisation that studies the medicine and social science of menses.

<www.cemcor.ubc.ca> The site of CEMCOR: Centre for Menstrual Cycle and Ovulation Research. A research centre with a mandate to distribute information directly to women about changes through the life cycle, from adolescence to menopause.

For good reading about girls reaching puberty and beyond

Jane Bennett, *A Blessing Not a Curse: A Mother Daughter Guide to the Transition from Child to Woman*, Sally Milner Publishing, Bowral, NSW, 2002. Available from <www.fertility.com.au> and by email: info@nfmcontraception.com

Amrita Hobbs, *Getting Real . . . About Growing Up*, Getting Real Books, Mullumbimby, Australia, 2003. Available from <www.amritahobbs.com>.

Shushann Movsessian, *Puberty Girl*, Allen & Unwin, Sydney, 2005.

Programs for girls and women

Jane Bennett offers these programs: *A Celebration Day for Girls* for eleven to twelve-year-old girls, *Cool on the Inside* for fourteen-year-old girls, *Fathers Celebrating Girls* for fathers of daughters and *A Blessing Not a Curse* for mothers of daughters. Contact by email: hijane@vic.chariot.net.au

Alexandra Pope offers the following programs for women: *Women Power and the Body*, *The Wisdom of Menstruation*, *From PMS to Power*, and a women's leadership program based on a woman's energy system. For nine to twelve-year-old girls and their mums: *Let's Talk Growing Up*, co-facilitated with Shushann Movsessian and Maree Lipschitz. Contact: genie@wildgenie.com

Shushann Movsessian offers one-day *Puberty Girl* workshops at Sydney's Royal Hospital for Woman, as well as at schools and privately; workshops for parents of pre-teen girls; train the trainer programs for counsellors, health professionals and teachers. <www.shushann.com>.

Amrita Hobbs offers *Girls Growing Up!* for mothers and daughters; workshops for women; *Rites of Passage* for teenagers, as well as programs in schools. <www.amritahobbs.com>.

Maree Lipschitz co-runs a corporate mothers program. For information email: menright@bigpond.com

Pathways Foundation offers *Pathways Into Womanhood*, a contemporary community-based rite of passage into womanhood, a five-day program for girls aged thirteen–fifteen years with their mothers or a woman mentor. <www.pathwaysfoundation.com.au>.

For good women's reproductive and general health information

Reproductive Choice Australia is a coalition of organisations and individuals who are interested in ensuring that women's reproductive rights are protected and enhanced in Australia. <www.reproductive choiceaustralia.org.au>.

The Jocelyn Centre for Natural Fertility Management and Holistic Health is a naturopathic and allied health clinic specialising in reproductive and hormonal health. Contact details above.

The following sites are also useful for women's health

<www.susunweed.com>.

<www.drnorthrup.com>.

<www.drclaudiawelch.com>.

<www.ourbodiesourselves.org>.

<www.westonaprice.org> The site for Weston A Price Foundation, an organisation dedicated to restoring nutrient-dense foods to the human diet through education, research and activism. It supports a number of movements that contribute to this objective, including organic and biodynamic farming, honest and informative labelling, prepared parenting and nurturing therapies.

<www.wddty.com> *What Doctors Don't Tell You* is a comprehensive review of health problems and safer, proven ways of treating them, as well as a place for you to share your health experiences.

<www.emofree.com> Emotional Freedom Technique.

<www.tftrx.com> Thought Field Therapy.

Alternatives to disposable pads and tampons

<www.radpads.com.au>.

<www.wemoon.com.au>.

<www.thenaturalcompany.com.au>.

<www.pleasurepuss.com>.

<www.mooncup.co.uk>.

ENDNOTES

Introduction

1 Barbara Seaman and G. Seaman, *Women and the Crisis in Sex Hormones*, Bantam Books, New York, 1977.

2 Quoted in Barbara Seaman, *The Doctor's Case Against the Pill*, Group West, Emeryville, CA, 1969, 1995, p. 2.

Chapter 2 The Pill is a drug

1 S. Siedlecky and D. Wyndham, *Populate and Perish: Australian Women's Fight for Birth Control*, Allen & Unwin, Sydney, 1990.

2 Reah Tannahill, *Sex in History*, Scarborough House, USA, 1992.

3 ibid.

4 Jerilynn Prior, 'Choices for effective contraception in 2006', <www.cemcor. ubc.ca> [3 October 2006].

5 Stephanie Paul, 'US likely to approve contraceptive designed to eliminate periods', *International Herald Tribune*, 19 April 2007.

6 Sherrill Sellman, *Mothers Prevent Your Daughters From Getting Breast Cancer*, GetWell International, Tulsa, OK, 2003.

7 Christine Read et al. (eds), *Contraception: An Australian Clinical Practice Handbook*, Sexual Health & Family Planning Australia, Ashfield, NSW, 2006.

8 John Guillebaud, *Contraception: Your Questions Answered*, 4th edition, Churchill Livingstone, Edinburgh, 2004.

9 David Lilley, interview, October 2006.

Chapter 3 The never-ending pregnancy

1 Andrew Coglan, 'How safe is safe?', *New Scientist*, 6403–43, October 1999.

2 Jan Roberts (ed.), 'The Pill and sex—risks to health and fertility', *The Foresight Association Newsletter*, Australia, 1995.

3 Kim Lai, 'The Psycho-Anatomy of Time', honours thesis, Deakin University, Australia, 1998.

Chapter 5 Feeling depressed?

1 World Health Organization, 'Mental health report', <www.who.org> [13 December 2006].

2 Jayashri Kulkani et al., 'Depression associated with combined oral contraceptives—a pilot study', *Australian Family Physician*, 43(11): 990, 2005.

3 Jayashri Kulkani, 'Depression link with contraceptive pill', <www.alfred.org.au> [28 February 2005].

4 'Inquiry into birth pill used to cure acne', *Daily Telegraph*, UK, 8 May 2006.

5 S. Robinson et al., 'Do the emotional side-effects of hormonal contraception come from pharmacologic or psychological mechanisms?', *Medical Hypotheses*, 63(2): 268–73, 2004.

6 A. Kubba, and J. Guillebaud, 'Combined oral contraceptives: acceptability and effective use', [review] *British Medical Bulletin*, 49(1): 140–57, January 1993.

7 C. Kay, 'The Royal College of General Practitioners' Oral Contraception Study: Some Recent Observations', *Clinics in Obstetrics and Gynecology*, 11(3): 759–86, December 1984.

8 S. Brunnhuber and S. Kirchengast, 'Use of the oral contraceptive pill by Austrian adolescents with emphasis on the age of onset, side-effects, compliance and lifestyle', *Collegium Antropologicum*, 26(2): 467–75, December 2002.

9 U.D. Rohr, 'The impact of testosterone imbalance on depression and women's health', *Maturitas*, 41: S25–46, April 2002.

Chapter 6 Low libido—is *that* how it works?

1 Lorraine Dennerstein, transcript from *Catalyst*, <www.abc.net.au> [20 May 2004].

2 Claudia Panzer et al., 'Impact of oral contraceptives on sex hormone-binding globulin and androgen levels: a retrospective study in women with sexual dysfunction', *Journal of Sexual Medicine*, 3: 104–113, 2006.

3 D. Blum, *Sex on the Brain*, Penguin Books, New York, 1998.

4 ibid.

5 Michael Richard et al., 'Volatile fatty acids, "copulins", in human vaginal secretions', *Psychoneuroendocrinology*, 1: 153–63.

Chapter 7 Mood swings, weight gain, brittle bones and migraines

1 P. Moro et al., 'Gallstone disease in Peruvian coastal natives and highland migrants', *Gut*, 46(4): 569–73, April 2000.

2   R. Burkman et al., 'Safety concerns and health benefits associated with oral contraception', *American Journal of Obstetrics and Gynaecology*, 190 (4 Suppl): S5–22, April 2004.

3   Jerilynn Prior, 'Choices for effective contraception in 2006', <www.cemcor.ubc.ca> [3 October 2006].

4   Jane Lyttleton, interview, January 2007.

5   A. Hobson and R. Grumman, 'Contraception secrets your doctor hasn't told you', *Cosmopolitan*, December 2003.

6   Siobhan Moylan, 'PCOS and the Pill', *Nova*, February 2006.

7   'Depot medroxyprogesterone acetate for contraception causes weight and fat gain in women', *Nature, Clinical Practice and Metabolism*, 1(69), 2005.

8   E. Diamanti-Kandarakis et al., 'A modern medical quandary: polycystic ovarian syndrome, insulin resistance and oral contraceptive pills', *Journal of Clinical Endocrinology and Metabolism*, 88(5): 1927–32, 2003.

9   B. Cromer, 'Bone mineral density in adolescent and young adult women on injectable or oral contraception', *Current Opinion on Obstetrics and Gynaecology*, 15(5): 353–7, October 2003.

10 Jerilynn Prior et al., 'Oral contraceptive agent use and bone mineral density in premenopausal women: cross-sectional, population-based data from the Canadian Multicentre Osteoporosis Study', *Canadian Medical Association Journal*, 165: 1023–9, 2001.

11 V. Beral et al., 'Mortality associated with oral contraceptive use: 25 year follow up cohort of 46,000 women from Royal College of General Practitioners' oral contraceptive study', *British Medical Journal*, 318: 96–100, 1999.

12 C. Cooper et al., 'Oral contraceptive pill use and fractures in women: a prospective study', *Bone*, 14(1): 41–5, 1993.

13 Jerilynn Prior et al., op. cit.

14 Karen Aegidius et al., 'Oral contraceptives and increased headache prevalence', *Neurology*, 66: 349–53, 2006.

Chapter 8   Dying not to get pregnant

1   R. Sachs et al., 'Reproductive mortality in the United States', *JAMA*, 247(20): 2789–92, May 1982.

2   Howard M. Shapiro, *The Birth Control Handbook*, St Martin's Press, New York, 1977.

3   'Venous thromboembolism & third generation oral contraceptives', <www.mhra.gov.uk> [3 September 2005].

4   H. Irfan, 'The Pill in Reproductive Management', <www.islamonline.net>
    [20 April 2006] republished from *Health and Science*, date unknown.
5   K.J. Pasi et al., 'Thromboembolism and the combined oral contraceptive
    pill', *The Lancet*, 345(8962): 1437, 3 June 1995.
6   Lara Marks, ' "Not just a statistic": the history of USA and UK policy over
    thrombotic disease and the oral contraceptive pill, 1960s–1970s', *Social
    Science and Medicine*, 49: 1139–55, 1999.
7   V. Beral et al., 'Mortality associated with oral contraceptive use: 25 year follow
    up cohort of 46,000 women from Royal College of General Practitioners'
    oral contraceptive study', *British Medical Journal*, 318: 96–100, 1999.
8   J.P. Baillargeon et al., 'Association between the current use of low-dose oral
    contraceptives and cardiovascular arterial disease: a meta-analysis', *Journal
    of Clinical Endocrinology and Metabolism*, 90(7): 3863–70, 2005.
9   Jerilynn Prior, 'Choices for effective contraception in 2006',
    <www.cemcor.ubc.ca> [3 October 2006].
10 C. Carter, 'The pill and thrombosis: epidemiological considerations',
    Baillieres Clinical Obstetrics and Gynecology, 11(3): 565–85, September 1997.
11 Ellen Grant, 'Cancer in a cream?', *What Doctors Don't Tell You*, 17(2): 6–9,
    May 2006.
12 ibid.
13 V. Beral et al., 'Oral contraceptive use and malignancies of the genital tract.
    Results from the Royal College of General Practitioners' Oral Contra-
    ception Study', *The Lancet*, 2(8624): 1331–5, December 1988.
14 ibid.

Chapter 9   On the Pill and pregnant—when the Pill fails

1   A. Kubba and J. Guillebaud, 'Combined oral contraceptives: acceptability
    and effective use', [review] *British Medical Bulletin*, 49(1): 140–57, January
    1993.
2   A. Hobson and R. Grumman, 'Contraception secrets your doctor hasn't told
    you', *Cosmopolitan*, December 2003.
3   Andrea Bonny, 'Weight gain in obese and non-obese adolescent girls initi-
    ating depot medroxyprogesterone, oral contraceptive pills or no hormonal
    contraceptive method', *Archives of Pediatrics and Adolescent Medicine*, 160:
    40–5, 2006.
4   B.G. Timms et al., 'Estrogenic chemicals in plastic and oral contraceptives
    disrupt development of the fetal mouse prostate and urethra', *Proceedings of
    the National Academy of Sciences*, 102(19), 7014–19, 2005.

5   'Women, contraception and unplanned pregnancy', study commissioned by Marie Stopes International, January 2008 <www.mariestopes.com.au> [9 February 2008].

6   B.G. Timms et al.

7   Francesca Naish and Janette Roberts, *The Natural Way to Better Babies*, Random House, Sydney 1996.

8   ibid.

9   'Oral contraception linked to prostate deformities', *New Scientist*, 3 May 2005.

10 Francesca Naish and Janette Roberts, op. cit.

11 Study: Mom's Pill Use Increases Boys Allergy Risk, <www.allergy.ivillage. com> [26 January 2007]; also published in *Allergy*, December 2006.

12 ibid.

13 Matthew Anway et al., 'Epigenetic transgenerational actions of endocrine disruptors and male fertility', *Endocrinology*, 147(6): 43–9, 2006.

Chapter 10   Off the Pill but where's the baby? When the Pill affects fertility

1   Francesca Naish and Janette Roberts, *The Natural Way to Better Babies*, Random House, Sydney, 1996.

2   Erik Odeblad and K Hume, 'Effects of contraceptive medication on the cervix', <www.woomb.org> [3 March 2002].

3   H. Irfan, 'The pill in reproductive management', *Health and Science*, reproduced on <www.islamonline.net> [20 April 2006].

4   Francesca Naish and Janette Roberts, op. cit.

5   E. Grueva and I. Borisov, 'The influence of chlamydial infection on the reproductive function in women with cervicitis', *Akush Ginekol (Sophia)*, 45(6): 35–9, 2006.

6   A. Khan et al., 'Correlates of sexually transmitted infections in young Australian women', *International Journal of Sexually Transmitted Disease and AIDS*, 16(7): 482–7, July 2005.

7   L.V. Westrom, 'Chlamydia and its effect on reproduction, *Journal of the British Fertility Society*, 1(1): 23–30, 1996.

8   M. Hassan and S. Killick, 'Is previous use of hormonal contraception associated with a detrimental effect on subsequent fertility?', *Human Reproduction*, 19(2): 344–51, 2004.

9   Francesca Naish and Janette Roberts, op. cit.

10   J.N. Lundström et al., 'Effects of reproductive state on olfactory sensitivity suggest odor specificity', *Biological Psychology*, 2005.
11   D. Blum, *Sex on the Brain*, Penguin Books, New York, 1998.
12   Sherrill Sellman, *Mothers Prevent Your Daughters From Getting Breast Cancer*, GetWell International, Tulsa, OK, 2003: 141.

Chapter 11 Malnutrition—a side-effect for everyone

1   A. Kubba and J. Guillebaud, 'Combined oral contraceptives: acceptability and effective use', *British Medical Bulletin*, 49(1): 140–57, January 1993.
2   Jane Bennett, 'Study of women's self-reported experiences on the Pill and other hormonal contraception: 1995–2005', <www.nfmcontraception.com> [15 February 2007].
3   ibid.
4   ibid.
5   ibid.
6   ibid., p. 185.
7   ibid.
8   ibid., p. 187.
9   Sherrill Sellman, *Hormone Heresy*, GetWell International, Tulsa, OK, 1997.
10   Andrew Weil, *Spontaneous Healing*, Ballantine, New York, 1995.

Chapter 12 Are periods really bad for you?

1   Elismir Coutinho, *Is Menstruation Obsolete?* Oxford University Press, New York, 1999.
2   Jerilynn Prior, 'Choices for effective contraception in 2006', <www.cemcor. ubc.ca> [3 October 2006].
3   ibid.
4   Stephanie Paul, 'US likely to approve contraceptive designed to eliminate periods', *International Herald Tribune*, 19 April 2007.
5   Jeremy Lawrence, 'Pill that ends periods sparks health row', *The Independent*, 4 May 2007.
6   Carol Tavris, *Mismeasure of Woman*, Simon and Schuster, New York, 1992.

Chapter 13 What about your teenage daughter?

1   Sherrill Sellman, *Mothers Prevent Your Daughters From Getting Breast Cancer*, GetWell International, Tulsa, OK, 2003.

2   Jane Bennett, 'Hormonal Contraception Survey 1997–2006' <www.nfm contraception.com> [2007].

3   ibid.

4   Jan Roberts (ed.), 'The Pill and sex—risks to health and fertility', *The Foresight Association Newsletter*, Australia, 1995.

5   F. Polatti et al., 'Bone mass and long-term monophasic oral contraceptive treatment in young women', *Contraception*, 51: 221–4, 1995.

6   *The Lancet*, 347: 1713–27, 1996.

7   D.B. Thomas, 'Oral Contraceptives and Breast Cancer', *Journal of the National Cancer Institute*, 85: 359–64, 1993.

8   *American Journal of Obstetrics and Gynaecology*, 1992.

9   Sherrill Sellman, op. cit.

Chapter 14   Taking the Pill for skin and period problems

1   Ruth Trickey, *Women, Hormones and the Menstrual Cycle*, Allen & Unwin, Sydney, 1998, p. 55.

Chapter 15   Are you thinking about coming off the Pill?

1   Francesca Naish, *Natural Fertility*, Sally Milner Publishing, Bowral, NSW, 1991.

2   Francesca Naish and Jan Roberts, *The Natural Way to Better Babies*, Random House, Sydney, 1996, p. 15.

Chapter 16   If not the Pill, then what?

1   John Guillebaud, *Contraception: Your Questions Answered*, 4th edition, Churchill Livingstone, Edinburgh, 2004, p. 48.

2   Gary N. Clarke, Scott G. McCoombe and Roger V. Short, 'Sperm immobilizing properties of lemon juice', *Fertility and Sterility*, 85: 1530–1, 2006.

3   John Guillebaud, op. cit.

4   ibid.

5   ibid.

6   Figure quoted from a conversation with Dr Kathleen MacNamee, Family Planning Association of Victoria, October 2005.

7   R. Butt, 'Men clamour to try out silicone alternative to vasectomy', <www.guardian.co.uk/medicine/story/0,1891798,00> [10 October 2006].

8   Francesca Naish, *Natural Fertility*, Sally Milner Publishing, Bowral, NSW, 1991.

9 S. Weintraub et al., 'Vasectomy in men with primary progressive aphasia', *Cognitive and Behavioural Neurology*, 19(4): 190–3, 2006.

10 Francesca Naish, op. cit.

11 R. Butt, op. cit.

12 Germaine Greer, *Sex and Destiny*, Picador, London, 1984.

13 John Guillebaud, op. cit.

Chapter 17 What are natural contraception methods?

1 Francesca Naish, *Natural Fertility*, Sally Milner Publishing, Bowral, NSW, 1991.

2 P. Frank-Herrmann et al., 'The effectiveness of a fertility awareness based method to avoid pregnancy in relation to a couple's sexual behavior during the fertile time: a prospective longitudinal study', *Human Reproduction*, 2007.

3 John Guillebaud, *Contraception: Your Questions Answered*, 4th edition, Churchill Livingstone, Edinburgh, 2004, p. 498.

Chapter 18 How to find the best contraception for you

1 Quoted in S. Siedlecky and D. Wyndham, *Populate and Perish: Australian Women's Fight for Birth Control*, Allen & Unwin, Sydney, 1990, p. 30.

2 Geraldine Matus, 'Are you managing your reproductive health care with informed consent?', *Femme Fertile*, <www.justisse.ca> [Winter 2006].

Chapter 19 Making the most of success rates

1 'Women, contraception and unplanned pregnancy', study commissioned by Marie Stopes International, January 2008 <www.mariestopes.com.au> [9 February 2008].

2 Leslie Cannold, on Late Night Live, *ABC Radio National*, Australia, 17 August 2006.

3 J. Guillebaud, *Contraception: Your Questions Answered*, 4th edition, Churchill Livingstone, Edinburgh, 2004, p. 13.

Chapter 20 What's the point of a cycle?

1 Deepak Chopra, *Restful Sleep*, Random House, Sydney, 2000, p. 12.

2 Maximillian Moser et al., 'Why life oscillates—from a topographical towards a functional chronobiology', *Cancer Causes and Control*, 2006, 17: 591–9.

3 Quoted in Sara Mednick et al., 'The restorative effect of naps on perceptual deterioration', *Nature Neuroscience*, 2002 <http://ernestrossi.com/ultradia.htm> [23 November 2006].

4 Jost Sauer, *Higher and Higher*, Allen & Unwin, Sydney, 2007.

5 Maximillian Moser et al., op. cit.

6 ibid.

7 Deepak Chopra, op. cit.

8 ibid.

9 Carl Honoré, *In Praise of Slow*, Orion Books, London, 2005.

Chapter 21 How to get connected

1 Black Dog Institute, <http://www.blackdoginstitute.org.au/depression/inteens/index.cfm> [23 November 2006].

2 Christiane Northrup, *The Wisdom of Menopause*, Piatkus, London, 2001.

3 Lara Owen, *Her Blood is Gold*, HarperSanFrancisco, 1993, p. 67.

4 Quoted in Ann Finding, *Anita Diamant's The Red Tent: A Reader's Guide*, Continuum International Publishing Inc, New York, 2004.

5 Quoted in Carl Honoré, *In Praise of Slow*, Orion Books, London, 2005, p. 14.

6 ibid., p. 117.

Chapter 22 Your very own feedback loop

1 Deepak Chopra, *Restful Sleep*, Random House, Sydney, 2000, p. 7.

2 Theo Colborn et al., *Our Stolen Future*, Dutton, Penguin Books, USA, 1996.

3 Quoted in Lynda McKewen, 'Social factors not hormones cause PMS, post-natal depression and menopausal stress', *Medical News Today*, 2006 <www.medicalnewstoday.com/medicalnews.php?newsid=45714&nfid=crss> [3 February 2007].

Chapter 23 Tapping your intuition

1 Sally Gillespie, *Living the Dream*, Transworld, Sydney, 1996.

2 Anita Diamant, *The Red Tent*, Allen & Unwin, Sydney, 1998, p. 193.

Chapter 24 Discovering natural calm

1 Carol Ann Raphael, 'Watching silence', *What Is Enlightenment?* <http://www.wie.org/j33/watching-silence.asp> [21 August 2006].

2 ibid.

3 Alexandra Pope, *The Wild Genie: The Healing Power of Menstruation*, Sally Milner Publishing, Bowral, NSW, 2001.

4   Sarah Buckley, *Gentle Birth, Gentle Mothering*, One Moon Press, Brisbane, 2005.

5   Natalie Angier, *Woman: An Intimate Geography*, Virago Press, London, 1999, p. 98.

Chapter 25 Getting high . . . naturally

1   Hal and Sidra Stone, *Partnering: A New Kind of Relationship*, New World Library, Novato, CA, 2000, p. 101.

2   Jalaja Bonheim, *The Hunger for Ecstasy*, Rodale Books, USA, 2001, p. 2.

3   Sarah Buckley, *Gentle Birth, Gentle Mothering*, One Moon Press, Brisbane, 2005.

Chapter 27 The natural way to menstrual wellbeing

1   Some information drawn from the Weston A Price organisation <www.westonaprice.org>.

2   Penelope Shuttle and Peter Redgrove, *The Wise Wound*, Paladin, London, 1989.

3   Tony Edwards, 'Wireless technology: something in the air', *What Doctors Don't Tell You*, 17(7), October 2006.

4   ibid.

5   Instructions for the Deer Exercise are taken from Lisa Bodley, *Recreating Menstruation*, Gnana Yoga Foundation, Melbourne, 1995 <www.recreating menstruation.com>.

Chapter 28 What *you* can do for your period and skin problems

1   Lara Owen, *Her Blood Is Gold*, HarperSanFrancisco, 1993, p. 83.

2   Joanna Evans, 'The low-down on low-fat milk', *What Doctors Don't Tell You*, 18(1), April 2007, p. 7.

3   Christiane Northrup, *Women's Bodies, Women's Wisdom*, Piatkus, London, 1995, p. 198.

4   Lewis E. Mehl-Madrona, 'Treatment of uterine fibroids with complementary medicine' <http://www.healing-arts.org/mehl-madrona/mmfibroids.htm> [accessed 5 July 2007].

5   Story taken from <http://www.wemoon.com.au/health_benefits.html> [accessed 25 September 2007].

6   Mark Hyman, email blog, [12 July 2007].

7   Joanna Evans, 'The low-down on low-fat milk', *What Doctors Don't Tell You*, 18(1), April 2007, p. 9

8 Jane Bennett, *A Blessing Not A Curse*, Sally Milner Publishing, Bowral, NSW, 2002.
9 'Acne and the Pill', *What Doctors Don't Tell You*, 13(4), July 2002, p. 7.
10 ibid.

Chapter 29 How your cycle is connected to your relationship

1 Judy Skatssoon, 'Do men cause PMS?', *Health Matters Features* <http://abc.net.au/health/features/pms/default.htm> 8 December 2005 [accessed 23 October 2006].
2 ibid.
3 Karen Houpert, *The Curse*, Allen & Unwin, Sydney, 1999.
4 Deepak Chopra, *Restful Sleep*, Random House, Sydney, 2000, p. 12.

Chapter 30 The slow route to a great relationship

1 Diana Richardson, *The Heart of Tantric Sex*, O Books, Alresford, 2003, p. 86.
2 Diana Richardson, *Tantric Orgasm for Women*, Destiny Books, Rochester, 2004, p. 30.
3 ibid., p. 29.
4 ibid., p. 23.

Chapter 31 Negotiating contraception

1 Harville Hendrix, *Getting the Love You Want*, Schwartz and Wilkinson, Melbourne, 1988.

Appendix 1 How the Pill does what

1 Christine Read et al. (eds), *Contraception: An Australian Clinical Practice Handbook*, Sexual Health & Family Planning Australia, Ashfield, NSW, 2006.
2 John Guillebaud, *Contraception: Your Questions Answered*, 4th edition, Churchill Livingstone, Edinburgh, 2004.
3 Christine Read et al., op. cit.
4 John Guillebaud, op. cit.
5 Christine Read et al., op. cit.
6 John Guillebaud, op. cit.
7 Christine Read et al., op. cit.
8 John Guillebaud, op. cit.
9 Christine Read et al., op. cit.
10 John Guillebaud, op. cit.

11 Christine Read et al., op. cit.
12 John Guillebaud, op. cit.
13 Christine Read et al., op. cit.
14 John Guillebaud, op. cit.
15 Ellen Grant, 'Cancer in a cream?', *What Doctors Don't Tell You*, May 2006.

Appendix 2 The Pill disturbs nutrition

1 Francesca Naish and Janette Roberts, *The Natural Way to Better Babies*, Random House, Sydney, 1996.
2 ibid.
3 ibid.
4 ibid.
5 ibid.
6 ibid., p. 185.
7 ibid.
8 ibid., p. 187.
9 Sherrill Sellman, *Hormone Heresy*, GetWell International, Tulsa, OK, 1997.

Appendix 3 What about a pill for men?

1 Sherrill Sellman, *Mothers Prevent Your Daughters From Getting Breast Cancer*, GetWell International, Tulsa, OK, 2003.
2 John Guillebaud, *Contraception: Your Questions Answered*, 4th edition, Churchill Livingstone, New York, 2004.

Appendix 4 Environmental side-effects

1 'Endocrine disrupting substances in the environment', *Environment Canada* <www.ec.gc.ca> [20 January 2005].
2 A. Black, D. Francoeur and T. Rowe, 'Canadian contraception consensus', *Journal of Obstetrics and Gynaecology Canada*, 26(2): 143–56, 2004.
3 C. Daughton and T. Ternes, 'Pharmaceuticals and personal care products in the environment: agents of subtle change? *Environmental Health Perspectives*, 107, Supplement 6: 907–38, 1999.
4 J.P. Nash et al., 'Long-term exposure to environmental concentrations of the pharmaceutical ethynylestradiol causes reproductive failure in fish', *Environmental Health Perspectives*, 112(17): 1725–33, 2004.
5 Theo Colborn et al., *Our Stolen Future*, Dutton, Penguin Books, New York, 1996.
6 B.C. Ryan and J.G. Vandenbergh, (in press), 'Developmental exposure to environmental estrogens alters anxiety and spatial memory in female mice', *Hormones and Behavior*.

7   Theo Colborn et al., op. cit.

8   ibid.

9   J. Raloff, 'Disposal concern focuses on wildlife —contraceptive patch worry', source unknown, [19 May 2006].

10 J. Raloff, 'Contraceptive ring could pose risks after its disposal', *Science News*, 163(4), 25 January 2003.

11 ibid.

ACKNOWLEDGEMENTS

This book has been birthed with the assistance of a fabulous retinue of helpers. To Francesca Naish, we warmly hug you for your integrity and dedication to health and fertility and your unbounded encouragement of our work. For generously sharing your time and professional expertise our heartfelt thanks go to Lisa Bodley, Cheryl Dingle, Wendy Dumeresq, Kaye Gartner, Mary Garvey, Sally Gillespie, Alastair Gray, Angela Hywood, Brian Keats, Dr David Lilley, Dr Jane Lyttleton, Dr Barbara Murphy, Geraldine Matus, Dr Ronnie Moule, Larry Phillips, Janette Roberts, Daniel Saulwick, Professor Roger Short, Claudette Wadsworth, David Wansborough and Dr Claudia Welch.

For a good couple of decades women have been telling us stories of their experiences on the Pill and of their journeys as cycling women. To you all: we are deeply grateful for your openness, generosity and excitement about this work. Without your stories we would not have known the full depth and breadth of the problems and issues, the pleasure and power that comes from valuing the cycle and, it's unlikely that the passion to write this book would have come to inhabit us so powerfully. While each story is unique and each has made an invaluable contribution we would especially like to thank Tania Anders, Fiona Barrie, Annette Baulch, Amanda Bennett, Kim Broughton, Autumn Brown, Marita Callanan, Lalita Claff, Elizabeth Hamilton, Stephanie Hamilton, Emma Hutton, Fiona Kane, Lisa Leger, Alice Masman, Karen Masman, Freya McIntosh, Lisa Mitchell, Fran Montague, Toni Pellas, Lindy Powell, Diane Riley, Victoria Royle, Melinda Smith, Blythe Tait, Jennifer Taylor, Helen Thomas, Paulette Tricarico, Nicole Tricarico, Jane Watson and Giri Wiseman.

We'd also like to acknowledge the many people who have gone before us in questioning the Pill, in particular Barbara Seaman and Dr Ellen Grant.

A very big thank you to Maggie Hamilton of Allen & Unwin who has so gently and wisely guided us through to a whole new experience of writing and articulation of our work—it's been very empowering. Thanks also to Alexandra Nahlous and Jo Jarrah for your great editorial skills and care, and Nada Backovic for your design flair.

From Jane: Thank you Freya for your enthusiastic encouragement and for helping us to see how it is for young women coming of age today. And thank you Kim for your great patience and understanding of the long, often invisible and chaotic process of bringing a book into the world.

From Alexandra: a special thanks to Amy Scully for your input over the last ten years. Your intelligence and commitment have been integral to the development of my understanding of women's cyclical power. Thank you to Shushann Movsessian for sharing your expertise about girls, and Maree Lipschitz for the fun and revelation we three have shared running our mother daughter programs. To Julie Cunningham, thanks for our stimulating conversations about women's power. I am also very grateful to Sandy West for your generous financial support and to Jenny Shanley for the design of the menstrual dreaming chart.

And finally thank you, dear reader, for it is *you* who gives our work meaning. Enjoy!

Permissions

The information on the nutritional disturbances in Chapters 9, 10 and 11 and Appendix 2 has largely come from Chapter 2 and Appendix 3 of *Natural Fertility*, by Francesca Naish, and from Chapter 7 of *The Natural Way to Better Babies*, by Francesca Naish and Janette Roberts, with their kind permission.

The story of Carmela in Chapter 4 has been reprinted here with kind permission from Fiona Barrie.

The 'Five ways to inform yourself' on page 132 has been adapted from the article 'Are you managing your reproductive healthcare with informed consent?' from *Femme Fatal*, Winter 2006, with Geraldine Matus's kind permission.

3939315R00180

Printed in Great Britain
by Amazon.co.uk, Ltd.,
Marston Gate.